A GUIDE TO ULTRASOUND AND OTHER CONTACT ELECTROTHERAPIES

A GUIDE TO ULTRASOUND AND OTHER CONTACT ELECTROTHERAPIES

and
Underpinning Science

Dr David C Somerville PhD CSci FRSA

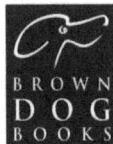

BROWN
DOG
BOOKS

Published under licence by Brown Dog Books and
The Self-Publishing Partnership, 7 Green Park Station, Bath BA1 1JB

www.selfpublishingpartnership.co.uk

ISBN printed book: 978-1-78545-271-0
ISBN e-book: 978-1-78545-272-7

Cover design by Kevin Rylands
Internal design by Andrew Easton

Printed and bound by CPI Group (UK) Ltd, Croydon, CR0 4YY

Acknowledgments

Thanks go to my wife Marjorie for her help and understanding as always.

Thanks also to TGS Electronics PTY, Australia and in particular to Scott Armstrong-Taylor for supplying equipment illustrated and used in experiments, and to Professor George Brown BSc DPhil D Ontology (Hon), FRSA for his comments in the preface.

Preface

This is the third text written on electrotherapies by Dr David Somerville. This one focuses primarily upon ultrasound techniques of therapy but also considers the more well-known TENS approach (Transcutaneous Electric Nerve Stimulation), the unusual method of shockwave treatment and the use of microcurrent therapy developed in the 19th Century. It also considers the potential of piezoelectrical transducers.

The text is well illustrated and informative. It does not shirk from providing technical details of the underlying physiological mechanisms which shape the processes of pain alleviation and inducing repair of tendons, muscle and other tissue. Each chapter focuses on providing understanding of these underlying mechanisms as well as providing data, references, uses in treatment and the limitations of the approaches.

Overall the book is a welcome addition to the literature on electrotherapies. It will be particularly useful to researchers and to those interested in deepening their understanding of why and how electrotherapies work.

Professor George Brown (Retired)

Medical Education Unit, University of Nottingham

Foreword

Dr David Somerville is the author of two previous books on electrotherapies. His background is varied from being electronics engineer to lecturer and medical researcher. He studied electronic engineering in the Royal Air Force, joining as a boy entrant at the age of 15. During his service he also studied industrial electronics at York. After a brief time employed as a research technician at Sheffield University, he Joined International Computers Limited as a peripheral systems technician but was rapidly promoted to senior engineering analysts, leaving after six years. After a short spell in project management at Marconi Space and Defence systems, he began an academic career by becoming a mature student initially studying physics, environmental chemistry and education subjects for 4 years. On graduation he became a college lecturer in electronics and computing whilst initially studying further for a master's degree as a part-time post graduate student in the Department of Orthopaedic Mechanics at the University of Salford. He graduated in 1991 after almost six years of postgraduate study, with a Doctorate in Orthopaedic Research specialising in fracture analysis. Postdoctoral supervision of PhD and masters' students led him to study non-invasive methods of stimulating bone growth and healing, particularly where non-union fractures occur, and similar methods of treating osteoporosis. He also studied 'Brain, Biology and Behaviour' for a year, along with 'Technology' with the Open University. Since 1994 he has been a consultant and international freelance lecturer. He also was a founder of The Institute of Registered Veterinary and Animal Physiotherapists (IRVAP). He was adopted into the name of Laycock, and many of his conference papers may be found on the internet under that name. He reverted to his birth name, Somerville, in later life.

Notes

Contents

Tables   **Page**

List of illustrations and photographs

Figure
1. Compression Waves
2. Transverse Waves
3. Ultrasound in water (photo)
4. Ultrasound head assembly
5. Absorption through various tissue types
6. Standing waves model
7. Ultrasound energy build-up
8. Reflected ultrasound energy
9. Longwave ultrasound in tissue
10. Pulse ultrasound chain example
11. Ultrasound tuning and calibration
12. Ultrasound equipment used in the experiment
13. Graph of temperature results
14. Diagnostic ultrasound reflection timing
15. Stylised representation of shockwave radiation
16. Neuron and axon formation
17. Typical action potential
18. Action potential conduits into muscle
19. Representation of striated muscle structure
20. Electron current flow along and through a muscle
21. Single polarity pulse chain
22. Biphasic pulse chain
23. Biphasic 'H' wave
24. Hall Effect simplified diagram
25. Direct current application to a fracture
26. Low-voltage attachment (equine photo)
27. Simplified representation of Gate Theory action
28. Logic circuit model - Pain Gate Theory
29. Gating theory of synchronous action potentials
30. TENS application alongside of the spinal cord (canine photo)
31. TENS applied to the hip muscles (canine photo)

Introduction

A definition of an Electrotherapy could be any therapy that derives it functionality from an electrical source. This may seem self-explanatory, but in fact refers to many modalities that require an electrical supply. The variety of therapy equipment could be covered by this definition includes such diverse ones as electrically controlled cryotherapy and heat therapies to radiation, induction and ultrasound therapies. In my own experience the main modalities mostly identified as specific electrotherapies for most veterinary and many human physiotherapists tend to be: ultrasound, phototherapy (LASER), pulsed magnetic therapy and direct electrical stimulation therapy including TENS. Sometimes these therapies are used alone or in conjunction with others alongside of the more usual hands on physiotherapy manipulation techniques. As we will see later in this book, research suggests that some tendon healing is best stimulated by a mixed application of phototherapy and shortwave ultrasound therapy. Pulsed magnetic therapy often supplements water-based therapies as does phototherapy.

In writing these books I have attempted to provide information for these modalities that helps the reader to evaluate at sufficient depth to not only understand the therapy but to be knowledgeable enough to explain the reason and effects of the application. It is hoped that these books will serve as a source of general reference for each of these increasingly used modalities. In this book I have referred to established research where needed to back up some of the text but in some other cases, have put forward original thinking and theories. These are exclusive and are open to scientific debate.

This is the third in a series of books by the Dr Somerville looking at specific electrotherapies. The other two being 'A Guide to Pulsed Magnetic Therapy and Underpinning Science' and 'A Guide to Phototherapy Practice Theory and Underpinning Science'. These books were written after many requests from both veterinary physiotherapists, students, and equipment owners to help give an understanding to the safe use and application along with the science behind these therapies.

This book covers the use of both longwave and shortwave Ultrasound used in therapy by giving explanations of both the application, technical and background to the development and use in practice. It also includes a shorter chapter on Shockwave therapy. The other treatment modalities include, electrostimulation, including faradic, TENS and microcurrent. This, like the others in the series, are written very much from a personal perspective based upon experience and background both in electronics and medical research. These books are not specifically written for their deep science and comparative analysis of relevant research, but to give substance to the science underpinning each modality. There are many well qualified people who research and analyse a wide range of stimuli that could be included under the common title of being an electrotherapy, however, for the student and therapist, this book should be used as a general reference to use in practice or for those who wish to learn more about the practicalities. Academic research of great depth may not have useful significance but where relevant to the discussions will be included. This book, like the others before, serves to provide sufficient knowledge to make an informed choice of the most suitable modality to treat specific conditions and understand any likely contraindications. Knowledge of the basic construction, functional operation, suitability and safe application of a specific electrotherapy is probably more relevant to the working therapist. The information provided in these books is aimed at assisting those without a deep scientific background to a level of understanding that can allow them to justify using electrotherapies to both the referring veterinary surgeon or medical practitioner. It also helps to be able to give an explanation where clients or patients ask why such therapy or technique in applying it is to be used.

Use of the term 'direct contact' in the title of this book refers to the therapies discussed within, in that they are applied directly to the skin surface of the patients being treated. Other therapies such as pulsed magnetic therapy, phototherapy and radiant therapies are applied near to but do not have to be exactly in direct contact with skin. They are very much electrically isolated and work by transduction into either photons, including those from within the visible range found from within a wide spectrum of frequencies up to x-rays, and gamma radiation levels, or by direct induction forming electrical charges in tissue from interactions with low-frequency dynamic magnetic fields passing through them. None of these require any direct electrical or mechanical contact. The direct contact of the therapies discussed in this book must necessarily be in touch with surface tissue over a precisely targeted areas to have any stimulation effect, or to enable a transfer of energy. A good knowledge of surface anatomy is assumed for the direct application of muscle stimulators to be able to apply and target specific areas of muscle groups to elicit a beneficial 'twitch' or contraction. With muscle stimulators or TENS stimulation for non-pharmaceutical analgesic they require a certain amount of skill before application. These establish direct contact by attachment of electrodes and are discussed in dedicated chapters.

Since this book covers several electrotherapy modalities, each one will be discussed in turn. The format will be to give background to the therapy, methods of application and then treatment conditions. These conditions, along with any risk or contraindications, should be considered when deciding on a course of treatment. As is usual in these books, information will be provided on the construction and the science underpinning each modality along with tissue reactions, effects and relevant research findings.

The first chapter deals with safety aspects and is a feature of each of my books. It is based on common sense approaches to safe use and application that should generally be applied to all electrotherapies. Direct contact electrotherapies come with additional considerations for safe application and the risk assessments to be applied. The format for the rest of the book will be sectionalised for each modality, starting with an introduction giving scientific background relevant to the therapy. It will then develop information about the modality that will help the reader understand function and application techniques.

Chapter One

SAFETY CONSIDERATIONS

In my previous books I have emphasised the need for safety when handling and applying any electrotherapy. The subject therapies of this book include devices and methods of application that can directly be felt by patients and, if not applied with care, can be the cause of negative reactions such as 'fight or flight' if incorrectly applied to both large and small animals. These are amongst several direct considerations to do with training and risk assessment but, in general, common safety practices apply to any electrotherapy device. This short chapter revisits some of the common-sense aspects alluded to in the introduction.

All previous books in this series include this section on safety. For readers who may have purchased the previous ones, I make no apologies for seemingly repeating certain common safety factors applicable to all electrotherapies. For readers who have purchased this book as a stand-alone, read on. For others, use this chapter as a refresher. Many devices are battery operated with low-supply voltages and generally few concerns in terms of electrical safety although there should some precautionary measures even when such low voltages are present. Since this text is written specifically for both ultrasound and direct electrical contact therapies then the need to take extra precautions are necessary, especially where some of the therapies require a mains supply. Ultrasound devices are slowly being produced to run from a battery supply but many of those still available for purchase are mains powered. This means that where their use is required in less than perfect electrically ideal situations, such as in stables, hydrotherapy centres etc., in fact their use anywhere where a damp environment may be present, extra care needs to be taken. Cables should be placed out of the way of horse hooves or animals such as puppies that may try to chew them. In the event of an animal, therapist or patient receiving an electric shock, disconnect the supply. If not directly possible, then knock off the source of the current with a broom handle or any non-metallic tool and, when secured, immediately seek medical attention. In the second book I went into further detail regarding risk assessment for the environment around. At the risk of being repetitive, remember to always be within earshot of another person and never work completely alone.

Ultrasound equipment may need servicing and retuned to match the applicator head after having extensive use. These should also be PAT tested (portable appliance tests) carried out by a specialist engineer. Following simple common-sense rules will make for a safe environment for all present including owner, therapist and patient. The emphasis so far has been on the veterinary use of equipment, but the same rules should apply to human treatment clinics and related treatment environments.

The safe working and operation of direct electrical stimulation equipment will be discussed in each of the chapters covering it. But it should be emphasised that for all the equipment that comes under the umbrella title of electrotherapy, users should be trained in its use to a high competency, especially if using such therapies in any professional capacity. Equally, owners of animals referred for therapy should ensure that those treating their charges are fully qualified to do so if they themselves are in possession or ownership of electrotherapy equipment.

Ultrasound, particularly shortwave, comes with extra risks if not applied properly. Internal tissue damage can quickly occur if the therapist or operator is not fully conversant with the therapy and the conditions being treated. Dyson M, (1987)[6] stated that "ultrasound treatment can only be assured if the user has a full understanding of the processes involved". It is for this reason that shortwave ultrasound and direct electrical stimulation equipment are not generally recommended to be hired out by the therapist for owners to treat their own animals, unless the owner is fully conversant with, and trained in its use, and is therefore aware of the risks involved. They should also agree to fully accept personal responsibility for any outcome. It is for this reason that to be able to successfully understand, use and apply ultrasound therapy, its construction, and science behind how it works and the contraindications to its use, that a major part of this book is written.

Another consideration for safety is that with ultrasound, whether battery or mains powered, it requires high voltages to power the applicator head. These high voltages are achieved by stepping up from the supply if a low-voltage battery source, or by transforming and processing the mains supply. Although some applicators, in their many forms, are designed to be waterproof and can be used, in certain situations, underwater, the control equipment is not waterproof and should be well protected. The cable connecting the control box to the applicator head carries the high voltage pulse chain to the head. Extra care needs to be taken to keep the cable in good serviceable condition and regularly inspected. With all good equipment any high-voltage pulses arriving at the head would be isolated from any mains supply, by a transformer at the output stage. This means that there cannot be any situation that earths the head breaking the closed isolation of the head by causing a circuit to the ground. All medical mains equipment should conform to: BS EN 60601-1:1990, BS 5724-1:1989. [25] Direct electrostimulation therapies should also be protected from any earth return to the mains supply, again by isolation as above. However, many electro stimulators are now powered by small low-voltage batteries.

Finally, electrotherapies should never be a substitute for prescribed medicines and diagnosis by physicians and veterinary surgeons. Also, ongoing prescribed medicines should never be discontinued in favour of any electrotherapy without appropriate consultations with the surgeon in charge of each case. Safety covers all aspects of electrotherapies including patient history, allergies and treatments to give optimum effect in both safe use and application.

Chapter 2

ULTRASOUND THERAPIES

Sound is a series of mechanical vibrations that are transmitted from a source through an intervening medium. It has all the elements required for energy transfer, these being frequency, amplitude and speed of transmission. The speed of transmission is a variable dependent upon the density of the transfer medium. This can be anything from gaseous, liquid or solid. It also can be reflected as demonstrated with echoes. The denser the medium the faster the transmission of sound energy. However, the absorption is inversely proportional. Denser mediums will dissipate, scatter or reflect the energy more quickly. Another variable that affects absorption is frequency. The speed of transmission through any specific medium of even density will remain the same for all frequencies applied to it. The velocity changes as the medium gets more, or less, dense. However, the transmission medium also attenuates at rates depending upon the frequency. Lower frequencies penetrate deeper than higher ones for all types of medium transited through.

In physics the wavelength λ (the time to complete one cycle) = Velocity/frequency or $\lambda = v/f$. This formula cannot be applied in general to sound waves as the velocity is not constant but variable and is dependent upon the density of the medium carrying it as discussed above. The terms longwave and shortwave therefore are generalisations of the proportionate wavelengths through similar tissues referring to low and high frequencies, respectively.

This book, like others from the same author, aims to discuss not just the therapies themselves but the science behind them. This includes how the equipment produces the different energy transfers to provide an all-round grounding of the subject. The level of science needed to understand this book is probably no higher than upper-school physics and biology. However, where explanations require an in-depth discussion of how certain of the electrotherapies interact with muscles, nerves etc. requiring deeper biological understanding, this will be discussed sufficiently to give an overall grounding of the subject.

Sound by general definition is that which humans can perceive. In terms of frequency, it ranges from the subsonic, that is lower than is normally heard by the human ear of around 15 to 20Hz, to ultrasonic above the human hearing range of 20,000Hz (20KHz) and beyond. In humans the ability to hear the upper end of the audio range reduces with age so the ultrasonic starting point is subjective. Ultrasound used in therapy is way beyond any human range, operating from around 40KHz up to 3MHz. The lower of these frequencies being called 'longwave' and the higher frequencies 'shortwave'. They use mechanical vibrations to transfer energy from specifically designed applicators into tissue to help achieve certain therapeutic effects.

In the physics of energy transfer, the amount transferred is directly proportionate to frequency and intensity. In the audible frequency band, sound at all frequencies penetrates human tissue such that at after certain high intensity levels it can cause an increase in temperature. The intensity of audible sound is measured in decibels (dB). This is a logarithmic scale from 0dB.

When used with sound intensities, 0dB represents a pressure of 10^{-12} Watts/m^2 (one micro-micro (pica) watt per square metre) this being the sound of internal body processes that is just discernible such as heartbeats, blood flow and air molecules physically colliding with the tympanic membrane (eardrum). The upper limit is 120dB representing a pressure of 10 Watts/m^2, this being the sound of a thunderclap at ground zero to the lightning strike, or a very loud pop concert. This upper limit is the maximum that the human hearing system can be subjected to for very short periods of time before permanent damage occurs.

It is referred to as 'the threshold of pain' although some references now set this at 130dB. Sustained sound intensities above this will cause permanent damage to the ears. Sound levels above the threshold of pain can also begin to cause other effects including increases in body temperature, bleeding from the eyes and nose and ultimately death. Extended exposure to lower noise levels around 90dBs can also cause cumulative damage to the hearing system.

The difference in pressure intensities between 0dB and 120dB is 1 to 1000,000,000,000. This is the incredible sensitivity range of the human ear within the audio band. The pressure levels used in therapeutic ultrasound is up to 4 Watts/cm^2 but are not generally transmitted through air as with audio sound but through direct contact and very localised. This will be discussed later in the book.

Sound frequencies can vibrate solids, liquids and gases, including those found within the body, the range and depth of absorption again depending upon the density of each medium and the frequency as mentioned. This is different to light and other electromagnetic radiative energy, where the speed of transmission is relatively the same for all frequencies with a miniscule slowing down, again dependent upon density as it passes through transparent materials. Sound, subsonic, audible and ultrasonic, varies in its speed of transit and very much depends on the density of the medium. The higher the frequency the quicker the absorption and dispersion of energy. This will cause damage when the energy absorbed exceeds certain thresholds. Unlike electromagnetic energy, sound energy at any frequency cannot pass through a vacuum.

With ultrasound therapy systems, transit through any solid or tissue is also dependent, as stated above, upon the density encountered, the frequency being used and the interface between applicator and targeted tissue. Application considerations will be discussed in chapter five. The physics of any energy transfer requires that there is a frequency (dynamic) component. Every part of the electromagnetic spectrum, apart from zero is dynamic. In the acoustic-mechanical range, sound at 0dB represents a minute dynamic quantity as, apart from in a pure vacuum, it is impossible to have a 'no sound' environment situation outside of a pure vacuum. This dynamic quality is measured by its wavelength or frequency. Sound waves form pressure disturbances in the air that radiate away from the source. If the source is an omnidirectional point, the pressure wave, under constant conditions, will follow the inverse square law. This means that it will diminish in intensity at a rate inverse to the square of the distance from that point provided that the medium is constant. Simply put, if measured at a distance 'd', then at varying distances of 'd', i.e. 2d, 3d, 4d etc., the intensity will be $1/2^2d = ¼$. $1/3^2d = 1/9^{th}$, $1/4^2d = 1/16^{th}$ and so on. This law is the same for radiation away from any multidirectional point source of energy and is a standard in all energy studies.

Sound waves, both ultrasonic and audible, can have two main properties based upon application these being longitudinal and transverse. Longitudinal are essentially pressure waves that compress and rarefy the distribution of molecules in sequence within the transmission medium as the energy is radiated away from the source. See figure 1 below.

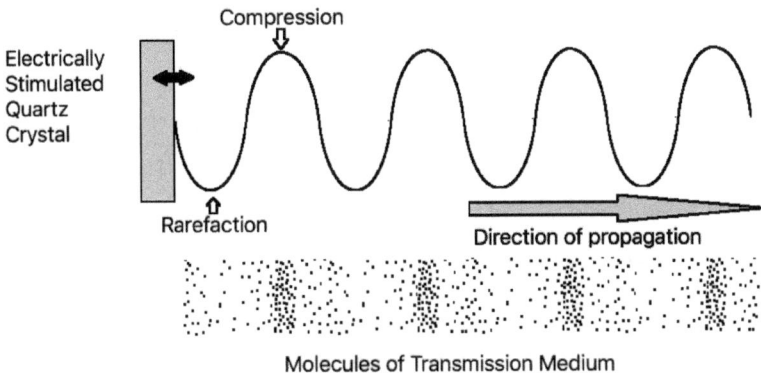

Figure 1 Compression waveform

In comparison to longitudinal compression waves, transverse waves effectively shake the medium from side to side. A simple example is the disturbance on calm water from a pebble being thrown into it. The energy of the pebble's contact with the water causes a point of disturbance at the surface that radiates outwards with the level of the water forming a transverse wave. See figure 2 below.

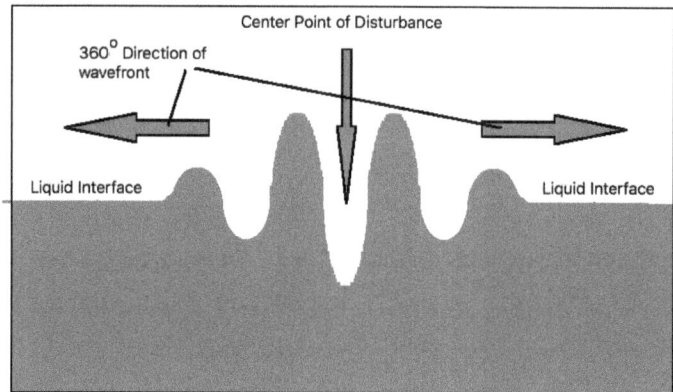

Figure 2. Transverse waves on a liquid.

In the above simple diagram, the waves would radiate outwards at 360 degrees from the point of disturbance, eventually forming a long-drawn-out damped oscillation until all the energy is dispersed. The point of disturbance will also form a central damped oscillation until the oscillatory level is again back at the zero level. The length between peaks under normal 'free' situations, is dependent upon the density of the liquid.

The use of transverse wave transmission is limited and may be of little use in therapy. However, some effect may be had when a pressure wave is applied to a hard structure such as the human tibial tuberosity. This may cause a transverse wave to be radiated as acceleration waves along the tibia at 90 degrees to the point of stimulation. This discussion will be added to in a later chapter where such effects may have significance to non-union fractures. Generally, from my own research I found that transverse ultrasonic waves propagate far slower than compression ones. With ultrasound and audio speakers the sound energy is more directable and is, under normal circumstances, composed purely of pressure waves. Both audio and ultrasound still diminish to a certain extent from such directable devices but are less widely dissipated, again dependant on frequency.

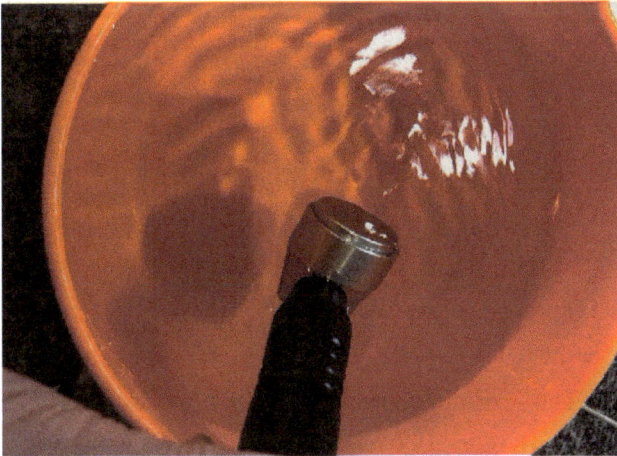

Figure 3. Shortwave transmission through water

Shortwave ultrasound, when radiated through a thin liquid such as water, can be observed to transmit in an almost straight line through the liquid with very little dispersion from a flat disc of the ultrasound head. This can be simply demonstrated with a bowl of water using a shortwave waterproof ultrasound applicator, see fig. 3 above. Also, it can be observed, with careful manipulation, that the beam reflects off the opposite side of the bowl in much the same way as an echo occurs in audible sound. This follows another physical rule that the angle of the incident wave will always equal the one being reflected. This quality of sound is important in understanding how ultrasound behaves when applied to materials with a high-water content, such as soft tissue, along with its ability to be reflected off internal hard surfaces. The latter may be the cause of some detrimental effects. The significance of this will be discussed in detail in chapter 4.

Ultrasound has many uses in the world where its ability to be reflected off interfaces within both solids liquids and gases is utilised. Modern ultrasonic car parking sensors are a good example of this ability as are those used in systems used to detect faults in structures by being reflected off the fault or crack forming an internal interface. This is a characteristic also used in imaging ultrasounds used in both human and veterinary medical diagnostics. Very short duration single pulses in the order of less than 1 microsecond, are transmitted from a piezoelectric transducer where sometimes the same piezoelectric transducer that initiates the pulse also detects the reflected pulses. If the speed of transit in the material is known, the precise location and depth can be calculated from the time taken for the reflected pulse arriving back at the head compared to when it was initiated. This is analogous to RADAR systems used in both aviation and weather detection. It is not necessarily the case that a hundred percent reflection of the ultrasound pulse is returned to the detector from denser internal tissue, some is absorbed by that tissue. In the case of imaging ultrasounds part of each pulse is returned but some carries on through to the next internal interface. This allows a more detailed structural image to be formed with further reflections and corresponding time intervals of the detected echoes.

The ability of shortwave ultrasound to travel in a relatively straight beam through materials with little dispersion is again the function of the frequency and the design of the applicator head. These characteristics found in diagnostic ultrasound have an equivalence to those used in ultrasound therapy with some specific differences in the way it is both transmitted, absorbed and in some cases reflected by interfaces within tissue, such as bones and tendons. Therapeutic ultrasound is, to date, probably one of the least researched modalities. Understanding the technicalities of how it is produced, applied and its possible tissue effects may help therapists and clinicians to make an informed decision whether to include it in their choice of treatment modalities.

Chapter Three

THE QUARTZ PIEZOELECTRIC TRANSDUCER

The title 'transducer' applies to any device that can transform one form of energy into another. The universe is observable because of transductions of energy and follows the law of conservation of energy. This states that the energy in any closed system remains the same being neither created or lost. This somewhat complicated statement simply means that energy is never really lost, just changed. The closed system is a theoretical entity as all energy eventually disperses through entropy, effectively ending up as heat. Any device that can change one form of energy to another is called a transducer. Everyday objects are transducers such as light bulbs changing electrical energy into light energy and heat energy. Electric motors change electrical energy into mechanical ones or in reverse changing mechanical energy into electrical energy. There are many other of examples of such transformations and a piezoelectric transducer utilising this specific quality of quartz is just one of them. These can transduce electrical energy into mechanical energy and vice-versa. Because of the high mechanical frequency of vibrations required in ultrasound measurements and therapy, these quartz transducers are currently the only forms of transducer ideally capable of providing the high mechanical vibrational frequencies used in ultrasonic therapies.

Speakers used to generate audible sound can reproduce frequencies of up to the limits of the human hearing range. Electromagnetic devices called 'woofers' and 'tweeters' are designed to efficiently convert electrical signals of both low and high frequencies respectively covering the full range. These are usually identified by being either large or small constructions. Frequencies much higher than 20kHz need other methods to transduce to higher frequency sounds, useful in both therapy and diagnostics and this is achieved through materials such as ceramic quartz where the 'piezoelectric' effect can be made use of.

The word piezo comes from 'piezein' (πιέζειν) which in the Greek language means to 'push'. Electric is from the word for amber (ἤλεκτρον) 'ēlektron' where in ancient Greece, attraction and clinging was observed between them when amber was rubbed with fine cloths. Nearly all crystalline structures including those found in bone structures (hydroxyapatite) have a piezoelectric property that plays an important part in bone maintenance and repair. Essentially, when a crystal is compressed some of the electrons making up the covalent crystalline structure are momentarily displaced. This forms a short-lived detectable charge across the faces of the crystal.

The use of quartz to generate electric charges is not new. Quartz pickups are still commonly used in some older record players where the grooves of the vinyl record carry the sound patterns. This vibrates the needle that is in turn directly connected to a crystal. They are also extensively used in electric guitars as the pickup transducers. The vibrations correspond to the sounds or music recorded as physical variations in the groves as the disc rotates or as the guitar strings vibrate. The quartz crystal produces a varying electric charge matching the sounds. Wires connected across the planes of the crystal transfer this charge that is then fed to an amplifier then onwards to a speaker.

This ability of quartz to be able to convert mechanic vibrations into electric charges can also be equally reversed. When an electric charge is fed across the opposite planes of a crystal it will momentarily change shape in the opposite way from that in which it generates a voltage. If the voltages applied to the crystal are repetitive and pulsed at a high rate, the crystal will vibrate at the same pulsing rate. This vibrating crystal can have such frequency and intensity that, if mounted in a specially designed head, can transfer vibrational energy to any medium applied directly or connected to it. This includes air at lower ultrasound frequencies. If the applied charge acoustically varies, then the crystal will respond accordingly and vibrate as the voltage changes. In the context of sound frequencies in the audible range, it can reverse the initial transduction and produce sound. This reverse transduction process was made use of in small crystal earpieces that can be still found around today. If a pressure is applied to compress the crystal and the pressure sustained becoming static, the crystal structure will return to an electrically neutral state.

When a compressive distortion is taken away, the crystal will return to its original physical state and in the process, momentarily produce a voltage across the plane in the opposite polarity to the one that was produced on compression. With electrical stimulation, maintaining a static electrical charge applied across a crystal will not keep the crystal deformed. Electrons will eventually return to normal distribution within the crystal structure maintaining an electrical neutral balance within that structure but there will be an opposite effect when the charge is removed. Each pulse of electric charge effectively produces a 'damped oscillation' that quickly peters out to zero.

Ultrasound transducers used in therapy are piezoelectric ones operating in the same reversible way as discussed above, but the main difference is that they are optimised by being cut and fitted to a suitably designed head that can be applied directly to target tissue. The size of the quartz is important as it will have its own mechanical resonance. Efficiency may be maximised if the vibration rate of 800kHz to 4MHz, for shortwave therapy application, matches this resonance or is a harmonic of it. However, driving it with a sufficiently high voltage chain of pulses may overcome the natural resonance to provide the desired pulse rate.

Longwave ultrasound uses crystals cut to maximise vibrations of around

40KHz. An electronically generated chain of sharp high - voltage pulses at the required frequency will cause the quartz to deform, effectively twitching. These individual physical twitches should each be of very short duration measured in microseconds and will occur when the electric charges are applied across the crystal planes. With shortwave ultrasound, if a stream of charges corresponding to a pulse chain of 1mHz is applied, then the crystal will physically vibrate at this same high -frequency rate.

The charges use to stimulate the quartz have to be sufficiently high enough to cause the intensity of the crystal vibrations to be of value in therapy or diagnostics. This means that the pulse chain applied must have a very high amplitude, corresponding to a voltage that is possibly over 100 Volts. In some cases, the electronics provides selectable pulse chains at three different frequencies to the same crystal. Provided that the physical twitch caused by each pulse applied does not interfere with the next one then it is possible to get a higher frequency range of outputs from one therapy head.

To transfer these physical vibrations into target tissue, the crystal must be mounted such that its connections from the driving electronics are fully screened and electrically isolated. If such units are mains voltage powered then they must follow safety regulations, again as stipulated in BS EN 60601-1:1990, BS 5724-1:1989.[25] These standards ensure that the contact head cannot form a closed circuit back to earth or the neutral connection of the mains supply. This is achieved by using a BS 5724 approved isolating transformer in the power stage to the head.

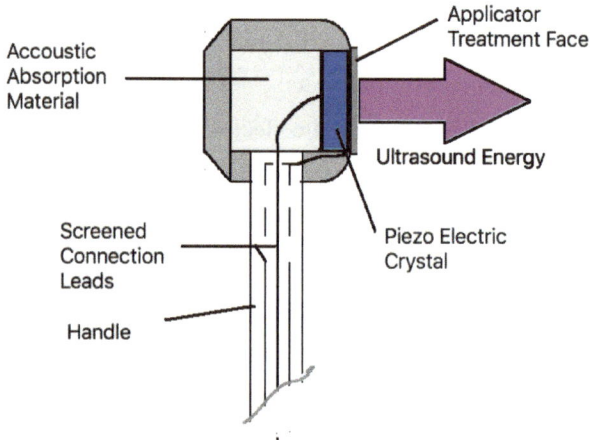

Figure 4. Ultrasound head assembly.

If a 1 MHz ultrasound head is operating and applied to soft tissue on relatively dry skin, then only a small amount of the energy available will be transferred into the tissue. This is because a mismatch of mechanical impedance at the interface. In electronic terms, impedance refers to the ability to transfer energy between two coils as found in a transformer. If the characteristic of the inducing coil and its circuitry matches those of the secondary coil in which energy is to be transferred, then a maximum transfer will take place. The same principle applies to that between a therapy head and soft tissue. Clearly the solid head of the applicator face is completely different to that of soft tissue such as skin surface. Therefore, to be effective, a way of matching the differences must be employed. This is usually achieved by a water-based gel or an electrical conducting gel, sometimes termed 'electro-gel'.

Because the gel effectively forms a barrier between the solid surface of the head and the soft target tissue by bonding to both surfaces it forms a common interface. The term 'thixotropic' applies to the shear quality of gels and certain liquids. This means that the gel will become less viscous when subjected to a rapidly changing force but returns to its normal viscosity after a short but finite time. The high-frequency vibration of the ultrasound pulses will lower the viscosity of the gel and keeps it low. The time between pulses is far shorter than the thixotropic rate of the gel. This means that possibly less energy is lost and the distance between the head and tissue is narrowed, allowing a greater transfer of energy. Up to 90% transfer efficiency is possible using specialised gels.

Using applicators under water is also possible providing that the equipment head is fully waterproof and is designed to allow it. Water acts as a coupling agent but quantifying its efficiency as a transfer medium is difficult. Shortwave ultrasound energy transits through water very easily as can be seen in figure 3. Its ability to be reflected can also easily demonstrated in the water experiment. This means that when water is used for coupling the head to tissue, a reflection is easily caused if the head is not tightly held in place. Water helps coupling but is not the ideal method although, as will be discussed later, it has been used in research with some success.

Chapter Four

ULTRASOUND ABSORPTION INTO TISSUE

Animal tissue presents varying arrays of density in both liquid and solid and a variety of soft tissues. Once an amount of ultrasound energy has entered the tissue several things will happen. These include: absorption, dispersion, reflection and attenuation. Other effects with shortwave ultrasound include stable and unstable cavitation, along with the possibility of thermal changes and cellular membrane potential changes. This chapter will deal with some of these effects and report on our own experiments using shortwave equipment and temperature measurements.

Table 1 below shows energy levels from ultrasound application at distances from the head in tissue. It is generalised, but not absolute, since within all three tissue mediums there will be variations. Hard tissue is not listed for shortwave but, with longwave ultrasound, it will absorb a large amount of the energy. Hard tissue such as bone can also form a very reflective interface to the high frequencies of shortwave ultrasound. This bony interface will largely block any onward transmission through it as it will be reflected. It is these reflections that play a part in the formation of unstable cavitation effects.

	1 MHz 50% Level	3MHz 50% Level
Fat	50mm	15.5mm
Muscle	9mm	3mm
Tendon	6.2mm	2mm

Table 1. Shortwave ultrasound tissue absorption

It can be deduced from this table (table 1) that the lower the water content of tissue, the greater the absorption taking place and hence, the less the depth of penetration. This may seem a slight contradiction as, with experiments using pure water, ultrasound beams appear to reach much greater distances than the above table suggests. It is the combination of liquid and solid tissue structures forming tissue that gives rise to the above table.

Water content is the important factor where it facilitates more efficient scattering of the ultrasound energy with reflections off shared tissue structures. This gives rise to apparently lower penetration depths. Muscle water content is given by various sources as 75% (see reference section) whereas fat contains only 10%. Muscle contains glycogen, a form of glucose storage, and it is this that is made up of 75% water. Tendon has a high collagen content that contains up to 60% water, but the greater absorption suggests that overall, it has a higher and more efficient scattering effect than muscle, possibly due to a more complex tissue structure. The table also shows that absorption is almost inversely proportionate to frequency applied, regardless of the tissue type.

Another factor in the absorption through various tissue types is the protein content of the tissue. The greater the amount of protein making up the tissue, the better the absorption. Figure 5 below shows the relationship to various tissue types and that cartilage and bone have the greatest absorption coefficient.

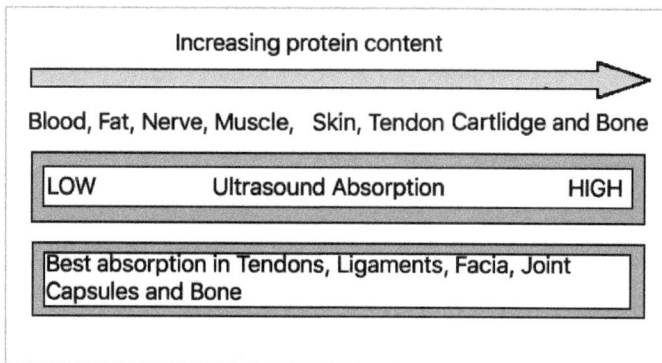

Fig. 5 Absorption through various tissue types

Absorption is also inversely related to the depth of penetration, as is frequency, meaning that high absorption equals low penetration and vice versa. Most references, as shown in table 1, suggest a depth of 3 to 5 cm for 1 MHz and 1 to 2 cm for 3 MHz. These figures are an average for all tissues, but fatty layers can conduct ultrasound to several times this depth. We have attempted to measure effective depth by both thermal imaging and direct temperature measurements. These will be discussed in the next chapter.

Another aspect of ultrasound absorption into tissue is the immediate effect of cavitation. This is divided into two types, stable and unstable. Stable cavitation is established within the first 1000 pulses, in other words, within 1 millisecond (1msec for a 1MHz beam). Cavitation is the production of bubbles from liquids within the ultrasound beam as it is absorbed into tissue. Since interstitial tissue has a large liquid content then the thixotropic effect caused by high-frequency ultrasound vibration will possibly cause a reduction in liquid viscosity and pressure compared to the surrounding tissue. It is this lower viscosity and pressure that may be responsible for the formation of micro- bubbles. Also related is the rarefaction pressure measured in pascals or more commonly MPa (megapascals) and which is a major contributor. The *Journal of Ultrasound Medicine* (2012)[12]suggests that the low pressure of just 1 or 2 mPa causes a rapid formation of cavitation where hard tissue is present. Rarefaction is the lower part of the ultrasound pressure wave, as opposed to the peak (compression). However the mechanism by which these initial bubbles are formed, they are said to have a therapeutic effect. It is suggested from various sources that it causes a sort of micro-massage. This is not substantiated in any research currently available. The action of this 'massage' may be due to the rate of overall formation and subsequent collapse of the bubbles and could be at a much lower rate than the frequency of the applied ultrasound.

With pure water, vaporisation can be observed by placing (for a brief time) drops of water on an active shortwave ultrasound head. The water is said to be 'atomised' forming a vaporised mist of water droplets. Atomising is a misleading term in terms of liquids but is generically applied to the breaking down of water into micron-sized droplets forming the mist. Although this demonstration is not within an enclosed system, this vaporisation along with the reduced viscosity may more readily cause the formation of droplets within tissue and the spaces between them to become the micro-bubbles.

Unstable cavitation is a problem mostly found in short wave ultrasound applications. It is in effect a larger build-up of bubbles that directly impact on tissue structures. These bubbles may be the same ones that occur within the first millisecond but begin to join making larger bubbles where the ultrasound waves are reflected off hard tissue structures. Having first passed through soft tissue and reflected along the same line as the incoming beam, they will then begin to interfere with that incoming beam forming hotspots and more bubbles. Standing wave formation may occur such that it will build up over a very short period of time to high energy levels thus causing these larger bubble formations to increase and also raising the temperature. The enlarged bubbles will begin to damage and displace tissue until they collapse potentially causing further damage to other nearby tissue structures.

Although the wavelength of ultrasound beams is variable, the wavelength is dependent upon the density of the tissue. In air sound travels (propagates) at around 330 meters per second (330m/Sec^{-1}). A 1 MHz ultrasound beam would have wavelengths of 330 / (1 x 10^6) meters in this environment. This equates to a wavelength of around a third of a millimetre. In tissue the density is greater than that of air, so the propagation speed is higher. Various sources including one from Georgia State University, referenced at the end of the book and found from a web search, suggests that around 1560 m/sec is a common value. The 1 MHz wavelength at this speed would be: 1560/ (1 x 10^6) meters = 1.56 mm. Subcutaneous tissue overlaying hard tissue such as bony prominences may be just a few millimetres thick and this is enough width to establish a standing wave.

To visualise what a standing wave is can simply be demonstrated by a tethered rope. Flicking the rope to send a wave along it will see it reflected from the tether. Flicking the rope at a constant rate will see the reflections interfering with the incoming ones such that, at specific rates of flicking, standing waves occur.

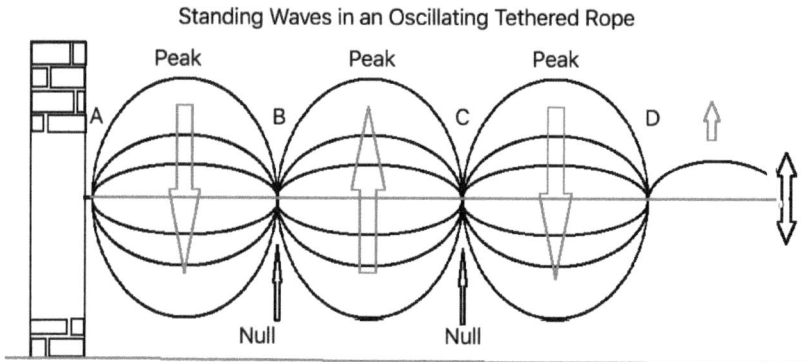

Fig 6. Standing waves model

It can be seen in fig. 6 that when a certain rate of these oscillations of the rope occurs, also called resonance, the rope will pivot about fixed points where the wave being reflected cancels out the incoming one. This pivoting point is a 'null' point. The peak points are where there is an additive effect at the high point as the maximum displacements of the two waves cross and add to each other. A, B, C and D in the above diagram correspond to the nul points. The distance from A to C or B to D would equal one full wavelength of the mechanical oscillation. If we compare the length of this rope in relative terms to the thickness of underlying tissue, it is obvious that an ultrasound standing wave can occur within a few millimetres of the ultrasound head if applied on thin tissue overlaying bone. It is in these cases that tissue damage can be most likely to occur when incorrectly applied.

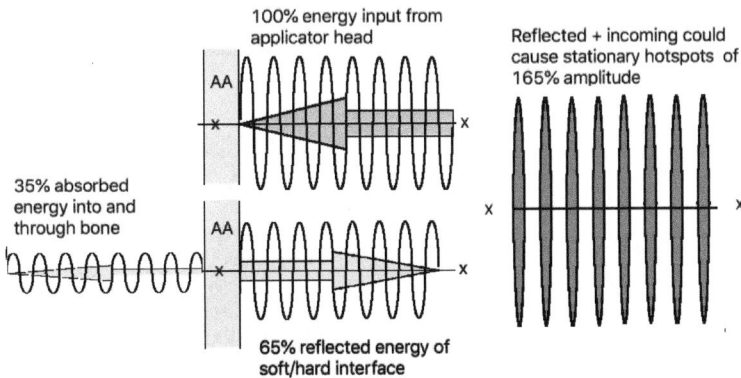

Figure 7. Ultrasound energy build up from a reflected wave.

Figure 7 above illustrates the build-up of ultrasound energy reflected from a soft tissue/hard tissue interface. This reflected energy is along the same line as that coming from the ultrasound head. Many references, including Nicholas D (1982)[17], give reflection coefficients between soft and hard bony interfaces as 65% meaning that only 35% is absorbed and the 65% reflected. Figure 7 was drawn for simplicity without any attenuation within tissue but shown as a reduction when reflected of the hard tissue interface. Energy passing through tissue along the line XX will be reflected along the same XX line from AA. The peaks of the incoming waves will then begin to add to the reflected waves causing a gradual build-up of energy thus becoming standing waves up to several times the initially applied level. If the applicator is held stationary allowing enough time to additively increase the intensity, this would effectively form those 'standing waves', as shown in the skipping rope analogy.

Fig 8. illustrates ultrasound energy passing through soft tissue and being absorbed (attenuated). As it is now being applied at an incident angle by gently being pressing at an angle into the surface of the soft tissue, the ultrasound beam will also be reflected at an angle back into the soft tissue from the hard tissue. Constantly altering the angles avoids energy build-up of standing waves and limits the possibility of unstable cavitation.

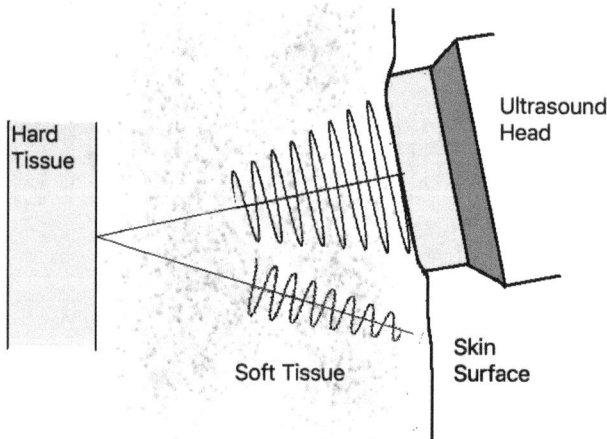

Figure 8. Reflected ultrasound energy within tissue

Longwave ultrasound of 40KHz would have a wavelength in air of 330/40,000 = 0.00825 meters. This equates to 8.25 mm. If the speed of propagation in tissue is the same as for 1MHz shortwave, then the wavelength will be: 1560/40,000 = 0.039meters or 39mm. Since the absorption into a tissue is inversely related to frequency, the lower frequency the better the penetration of tissue structures. Hard tissue such as bone can better absorb longwave ultrasound and so very little energy is likely to be reflected. Also, because of the longer wavelength, the room to establish a standing wave is very limited, so even if there is some reflected energy unstable cavitation is not thought likely to occur. See Fig 9 below.

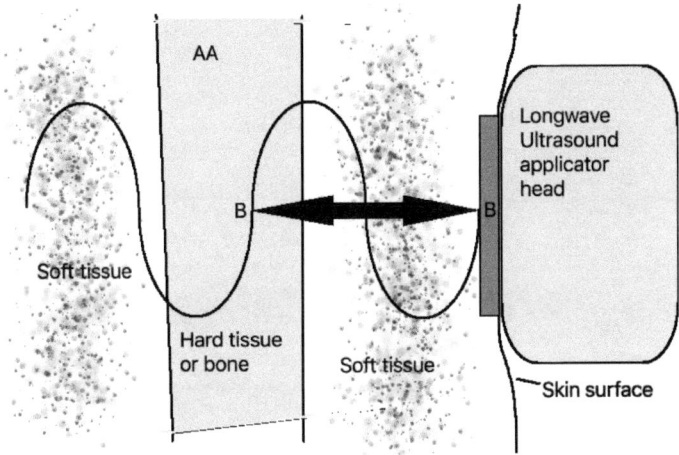

Figure 9. Longwave ultrasound in tissue.

The above diagram (Fig.9) highlights several points. Like a previous simplified diagram in fig. 7, it does not show attenuation in either hard or soft tissue, but it does show the relationship between wavelength, B to B, and the depth of tissue it passes through until encountering bone or other harder tissue (AA). With the energy waveform travelling in the direction indicated by C, the distance between the point of application to the interface AA is less than one wavelength. Since only a very small proportion of the already attenuated waveform would be reflected, it is highly unlikely that any standing wave would be established for long enough to cause cavitation tissue damage. The depth used to illustrate the above soft tissue is, in the real-life situation, likely to be much less than the 37.5mm wavelength. This means that the chance of cavitation is probably even less than discussed above.

Chapter Five

APPLICATION OF ULTRASOUND, THERAPY AND BIOLOGICAL EFFECTS

In the introduction to this book, safety was a major consideration both in terms of equipment safety and application. This chapter will look at the safe application of ultrasound therapy and compare shortwave and long wave types. The next chapter will concentrate on Longwave. This chapter will include discussions on the effects of ultrasound on the biochemistry and physiological effects offering some possible explanations and reasoning for such effects.

In the last chapter, the reasoning for the use of an ultrasound coupling gel was introduced. It was shown to be essential to allow a maximum transfer of energy and to lubricate the target area. This avoids friction of the head against the skin when applying movement to the applicator. This movement is essential when applying shortwave ultrasound not only to mitigate the possibility of unstable cavitation (see below) but to treat a larger area of target tissue. Unstable cavitation can also be reduced by pulsing the beam. All therapeutic shortwave ultrasound equipment should offer this facility. Sometimes the equipment manufacturer may offer different rates which can pulse the beam, but in general the settings are fixed.

Pulse Chain Applied to the Treatment Head

| 1 or 3 MHz | | 1 or 3 MHz | | 1 or 3 MHz | | 1 or 3 MHz |

Pulse Chain   On   Off   On   Off   On   Off   On..........

50% on 50% off Mark Space Ratio at Variable Pulsing Rates

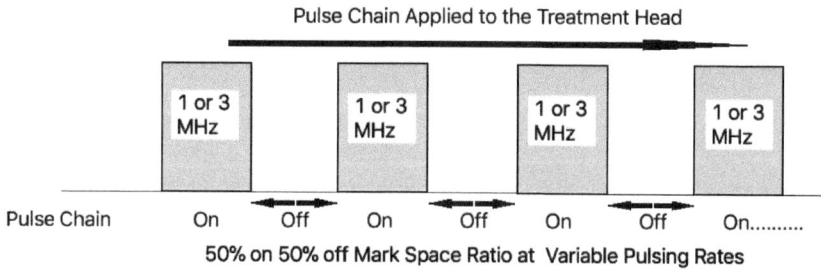

Figure 10. Pulse chain example.

With shortwave ultrasound equipment, the settings usually give a frequency (if multiple ones are included), with power levels shown in Watt/cm^2 and the option to pulse the output at around 10 pulses or less per second. The research findings of using pulsed settings will be discussed later. Pulsing shortwave ultrasound is also useful in that it reduces any heat build-up as greatly reduces or may even stop unstable cavitation bubble formation.

Stable cavitation will still form when using pulsed shortwave ultrasound since its establishment time is likely to be far shorter than a timed pulse of energy. The rate of pulses will have a probable mark/space ratio of 50/50 as shown in figure 10. The time to establish a standing wave in tissue requires a constant beam to be reflected off hard tissue back along the same plane as the initial beam being applied. Pulsing severely disrupts this reflected beam and possibly desynchronises it with the initial beam. The net effect is to inhibit standing wave and formation hence unstable cavitation.

At this point in the chapter it may be interesting to state that, apart from frequency, ultrasound pressure waves exhibit a reactive mechanical force away from the pressure head in line of the beam. When the heads need 'tuning' to match pulsed frequency from the driving unit, this is achieved in a tuning tank.

This is comprised of a square jar containing water, preferably deionised and bubble free, and a calibration lid comprised of a deflection plate assembly directly pivoted and coupled to an outside pointer. This points to a scale in Watts printed on the side of the jar. See diagram below in figure 11. The ultrasound head is placed through an access hole in the lid and is held in place perpendicular to and pointing at the deflector plate.

When the head is activated the beam strikes the plate causing a deflection. This deflection is directly proportionate to the energy level applied to the head. The directly coupled pointer indicates energy being absorbed on the externally marked and calibrated scale power levels. The equipment output is fine-tuned until the maximum deflection occurs. This method of fine-tuning of the head illustrates that there is a physical pressure exerted away from the head proportionate to energy output levels from the head. Because the beam is a series of high-frequency pulses, the deflection is an aggregate of the amount hitting the deflection plate. This pulsating force may form the basis of a physical micro-massage effect in tissue, especially if the beam itself is gated.

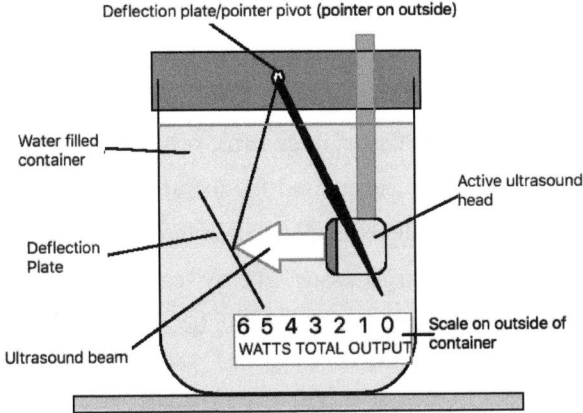

Figure 11. Ultrasound tuning and calibration tank system

Constant movement

By constantly rotating the head against the target tissue whilst maintaining full contact, cavitation cannot easily become established. Should hard tissue reflect the beam, it will be reflected through an infinite number of angles. The only problem that may occur is where the energy level is set high and applied to thin tissue covering bony prominences. There may not be enough room to angle the head and reflections may be doubly reflected to the applicator head leading to a rapid energy build up.

With longwave ultrasound, cavitation problems that may occur with shortwave ultrasound, are largely non-existent. With the physics of energy transfer it is the frequency that carries the energy. This simply means that the higher the frequency, the higher the energy that it carries and can transfer into tissue, but it is far more quickly absorbed and hence the depth of penetration is reduced. As a result, there is a higher energy density in a shorter distance than with longwave ultrasound. Longwave carries proportionately less energy density but has a far greater ability to penetrate tissues so that there are fewer reflections from biological interfaces including bone. Cavitation is therefore less likely to happen, as previously discussed.

Research carried out for the American Heart Association [1]found that, with 40kHz ultrasound, the energy through a pig's ribcage attenuated by 50% for each centimetre, but through soft tissue, in general, very little attenuation occurred. Since absorption into tissue is required for therapeutic effects to take place, the greater the absorption rate, ergo attenuation through target tissue, the more energy is absorbed by that target tissue. Energy scattering is a characteristic of all varieties of energy transfer. This above can be summarised by:

Shortwave Ultrasound

Higher frequency, greater scattering, less depth of penetration, has potential to cause unstable cavitation.

Longwave Ultrasound

Lower Frequency, less scattering, greater depth of penetration. Far Less likely to cause, if any, cavitation.

It has long been suggested that the primary effect of any ultrasound when applied to tissue is thermal. As long ago as 1953 Lehmann [14] used it as 'mechanism' for tissue heating. Agitation through high-frequency vibration of tissue at high frequencies, may cause friction between tissue structures at the cellular level resulting in heat generation. This could relate to the term micro-massage discussed, although there is no research evidence that this is so at this time. However, it has been my personal experience that this general increase in temperature does indeed rapidly occur in practice and can be damaging.

A chiropodist used ultrasound in her practice on a patient's foot. She obtained a new shortwave 1 MHz unit and was unfamiliar with the output levels. After using it on a new patient she complained that she had caused a burn on the unfortunate individual and blamed the equipment. Asked to investigate, I found that this person had had no training in the use of ultrasound, had clearly not read the instruction booklet provided and had set to nearly the highest constant output level for the treatment. Safety assessment had not been considered or its possible effects within such a high concentration of bones as superficially found in the foot. The net effect would have been a quick build-up of unstable cavitation and heat resulting in a thermal hotspot and subsequent blister formation.

Thermal effects other than those caused by unstable cavitation can be beneficial, in that as a natural homeostatic reaction, increasing blood flow to the treated area would follow a temperature increase. At $40 - 45°C$, hyperaemia will result. This can be very therapeutic. The conditions that may benefit from hyperaemia (increased localised blood flow) may be areas of swelling as increased capillary blood flow opens the capillary fenestrations and perhaps relaxes true capillary sphincter muscles. This allows a transfer of serum and blood cells both in and out of tissue. Initially, it may increase lymph flow as this is dependent upon hydrostatic pressure being greater outside of the lymph vessel to cause an inflow into it. Relaxation of tissue may also occur as an effect due to slight temperature increases reducing blood pressure. Increased temperature may help in the reperfusion of superficially accessible internal organs where ultrasound is safe to use.

For the purposes of this book a simple experiment was set up using short wave ultrasound applied to a section of shoulder pork. The temperature was taken at approximately 2cm depth by a thermocouple temperature gauge. With coupling gel applied over the area, the ultrasound head held tightly to the skin of the pork without any rotating movement being carried out.

Prior to the experiment both the pork and the ultrasound head were acclimatised to the local temperature of around 20C. This avoided the cold head of the applicator affecting the results and provided the base level for each series of the temperature readings. These were taken at 30-second intervals. The experiment was further repeated three times, starting with the unit set to 1Watt/cm^2 and then repeated with 2 and 3watts/cm^2 respectively, each at different points along the skin surface.

The following table shows the results.

Sampling time versus applied power	Temp °C at Power setting 1W/cm²	Temp °C at Power setting 2W/cm²	Temp °C at Power setting 3W/cm²	Temps °C at Power setting 3W/cm²
	A	B	C	D
0	20	19	19	22
30	21	24	35	25
60	21	24	40	25
90	22	24	41	26
120	23	25	41	27
150	23	25	43	28
180	23	25	45	29

Table 2. Experimental temperature measurements

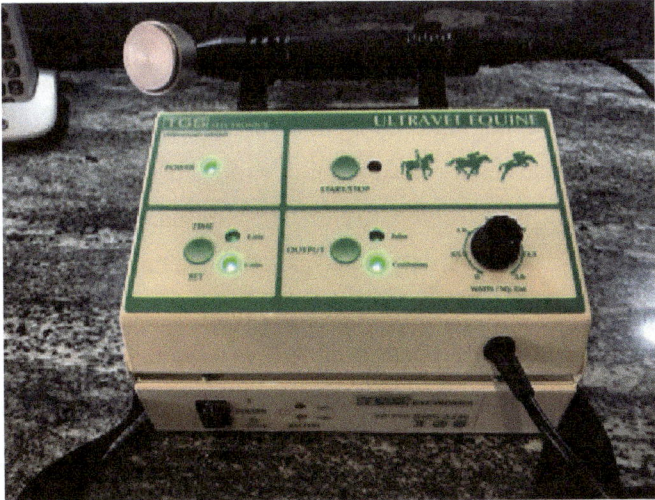

Figure 12. Ultrasound equipment used in this experiment

The above ultrasound unit had a maximum output power rating of 3 Watts/cm^2. The ultrasound applicator head measured a diameter of 3 cm. From πr^2 or $\pi(d/2)^2$ = area, this gives a total contact area of 7.068cm^2. The maximum ultrasound energy available was 3 x 7.068 = 21.204 Watts.

Columns A, B and C show temperature readings taken at different locations through the pork with similar depth of fat overlaying muscle at different power levels. The fourth column (D) was taken through a thick layer of fat but still at 2cm depth. This is shown in blue on Fig 13. All the readings confirm the fact that a major aspect of shortwave ultrasound is temperature increase. Results obtained from the 1 Watt/cm^2 appeared to show a modest temperature increase of 3^{0}C over a period of 3 minutes. This was similar at 2Watts/cm^2 again showing a modest rise only increasing the temperature by just over an extra 1^{0}C compared to 1 Watt/cm^2 over the full 3 minutes. Power levels set at 3Watts/cm^2 (green Fig 13) shows the most dramatic rise, increasing the temperature by 16^{0}C in the first 30 seconds. This rapid increase begins to slow down but still shows a continuous increase over 3 minutes.

Possibly the most interesting fact is the temperature change through fat (blue Fig 13) without any intervening muscle to alter absorption rates. Table 5, in chapter 4, represented the absorption in various tissue. Blood and fat were the lowest. This means the ability to allow the ultrasound energy to penetrate is the highest with very little absorption to pass through fat as shown by the graph in that although there is a rise of 2^{0}C in the first 30 seconds the subsequent increase over the next 150 seconds is modest, even though the energy level is at the highest for this experiment. A simple graphical representation of the above table is shown below.

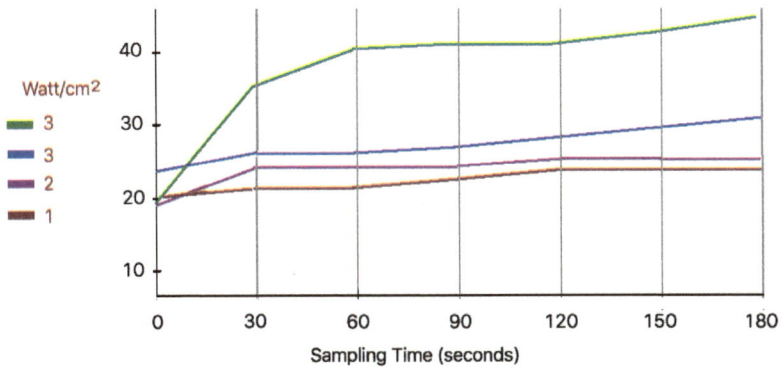

Figure 13. Graph of temperature results

The above experiment could have been improved in many ways and it should be borne in mind that in the living animal tissue the starting temperature will already be around 37°C. How much the applied ultrasound would increase this temperature in living tissue is speculative but may be proportionate to the higher starting point adding to this initial temperature in much the same ways as with the experimental 20°C starting point. This experiment was carried out to simply illustrate the thermal qualities of short wave ultrasound. Three of the sets of measurements were taken beyond the subcutaneous fat layer 2cm into the tissue. The fat layer was around 1cm thick. Where the fourth set of readings (D) were taken the fat layer was over 2cm. To establish hyperaemia this experiment suggests that, if the same increases in vivo are proportionate, the higher power levels are needed to cause hyperaemia. However, heat losses from the side of our sample tissue to air would reduce the overall and possibly slow down the rate of temperature increase.

Another consideration was the static nature of the ultrasound head in this experiment. In practice this would obviously have been circled to avoid cavitation. In this experiment the only interfaces were between fat and muscle tissue layers. It is unlikely that cavitation would have been established from soft tissue interface reflections.

Other temperature research with shortwave ultrasound

Research by Levine[16] (2001) carried out temperature measurements on live animals taken in the caudal thigh region. He used 3.3MHz on two different settings of 1 and 1.5Wcm^2. The depths of sampling were 1, 2, and 3cm levels with fine needle thermistors inserted and 10 dogs were used in the research. The applicator head size was smaller than our experiment, being 5cm^2. Overall temperature changes were after 10 minutes application were 3°C at 1cm depth into tissue, dropping down to 1.6°C at 3cm. This compared with 4.6°C down to 2.4°C at 1 and 3cm depths, respectively. Although this used a more concentrated head than our experiment and three different depths were tested, it confirms that at the lower power intensities a modest rise can be expected. A like-for-like comparison with our experiment is difficult as discussed in that the starting temperature on a live subject is much higher than our cold and raw pork sample. The validity of our simple experiment is valid given the reduced parameter of frequency, time and increased head size.

Other with treatments human patients suggest that applying to chronic conditions around joints may reduce swelling from within joint capsules but never during the acute phase of any injury, although the Minnesota Chiropractic and Rehabilitation Group suggest using it under certain circumstance due to it causing the release of histamines. Although no explanation as to why this should occur is given, it may be that acute tissue injuries naturally release histamines along with prostanoids through the damaged membranes of injured cells. The latter are more associated with chronic pain sensations. Ultrasound may raise the temperature around acutely injured areas and, because of thermal effect, potentially slow down the process of the natural closure and sealing of the phospholipid bilayers of the membrane causing further releasing histamines from cell cytosol. The suggestion is that histamines attract neutrophils and monocytes to the area helping to clear the area of foreign substances thus helping optimise overall healing.

Swelling may also be a chronic by-product of tendon injuries and this is where ultrasound finds a major use being both in the reduction of any swelling and as a stimulus in initiating healing of any tears or rips in the tendon. Scar tissue is problematic in both muscle and tendon injuries and is caused by unaligned collagen build-up forming in the affected area. In an area where tendon or muscle fibres need to align, the formation of unaligned collagen can be a cause of movement disorders in that collagen can resist tensile forces. Ultrasound has been shown to realign tendon fibres during healing and recovery. The scientific reasoning for this realignment is never really given satisfactory explanation. A possible one may be that the ultrasound waves cause an even scattering of tendinocytes through mechanical agitation. This more even distribution around an injury site may cause a more natural alignment of the collagen fibres within the tendon during the healing phase.

Benefits and Contraindications to using Ultrasound Therapy.

Using ultrasound therapy comes with some risks if applied to certain established medical conditions. Assessment of possible contraindicated situations requires a full history of any condition to be treated. Although many reports suggest various effects such as pain reduction, the initial cause of the pain needs to be known and possible underlying condition contributing to it. With soft tissue injury, damage cellular structures making up that tissue, releases prostanoids from within cell cytosol. This is caused by the rupture of cellular phospholipid bilayers forming the cellular membranes as discussed above. This in turn causes the leaking out prostaglandin that is produced within the cells.

Prostaglandin is a neurotransmitter that stimulates type C sensory nerve endings sending chronic pain signals to the brain, although ultrasound applied to an injured area may cause hyperaemia that is beneficial to the injury and help stimulate natural healing processes. It may have further benefits in that it may quickly disperse prostaglandin and therefore reduce its ability to stimulate chronic pain sensors by potentially weakening or diluting it. This in turn may reduce prostaglandin's ability to connect sufficiently to nerve ending receptors reducing chronic action potentials transmitted. This could result in either totally inhibiting chronic pain sensations or greatly reducing them. However, if the condition also is part of an injury such as a fracture then other method of pain reduction should be applied as ultrasound is generally contraindicated for healing fractures.

Applying ultrasound around a healing fracture may cause, in the initial post-fracture trauma, extra bleeding producing a larger haematoma to form than normal. This may be due to the thermal effect resulting in dilated blood vessels in adjacent tissue. Similarly, with developing orthopaedic growth, application of short wave ultrasound around growth plates is also generally contraindicated. In these cases, care must be taken when any required application on muscle groups is needed in areas close to young joints.

Regarding the above contraindication on young patients still developing long bone growth, Fréz[7] et al (2006) carried out research that applied continuous 1MHz ultrasound laterally to the growth plates of young rabbits. The amount of energy set was 1 Watt/cm^2 and applied using water as a coupling agent. His research suggests that it causes a possible disturbance resulting in damage to growth plates. The rabbits were two-month old when subjected to a five-minute treatment laterally to the right knee joint. They were treated for 10 days. The left knee joint on each of the subjects was used as a control. Histological analysis showed a 24.4% increase in thickness of the treated joints. Among the conclusions is that ultrasound causes an acceleration in growth plate metabolism. This would possibly cause developmental problems as the growth plates eventually calcify. The suggestion from the above research is that growth plate metabolism has significance in the use of shortwave ultrasound in stimulating mesenchymal stem cells producing cartilage.

Acute infections are also contraindicated, possibly for the same reasons as with other electrotherapies. Any electrotherapy that can cause an increase in blood flow may spread an infection to other areas of the body. Pulsed magnetic therapy may cause increased capillary flow. Red light phototherapy causes localised production of nitrous oxide from cyclooxygenase reactions. This in turn causes vasodilation of smooth muscle blood vessels. Since a reaction to localised heat effect from shortwave ultrasound also stimulates blood vessel dilation, the same spreading of bacterial pathogens would follow. The same logic could apply to other conditions where increased blood flow would normally be contraindicated. Typical conditions are those such as acute ischaemic tissue and conditions where there is a possibility of haemorrhage.

Ultrasound diagnostic equipment is used to examine developing foeti and has very few side effects. Ultrasound used in therapy is most definitely contraindicated for application anywhere near a foetus. As discussed in chapter one, diagnostic ultrasound is sent out in singular pulses that are insufficient to cause a rise in temperature or cavitation. These pulses reflect from internal interfaces and are mechanically scanned. The pulses are up to 3MHz in frequency and gated such that the time between a pulse being transmitted into the tissue has time to allow reflection to the ultrasound head from the deepest structure. Since each structure including a foetus may return a reflected pulse, multiple pulses are returned and detected by the scanning ultrasound head.

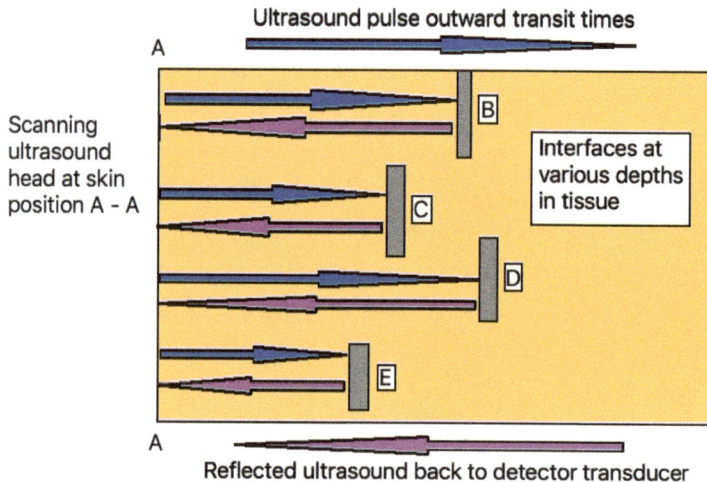

Figure 14. Diagnostic ultrasound reflection timing

Figure 14 is a simple illustration of timing. Pulse A enters the tissue and takes differing amounts of time to reach and then be reflected off different tissue interfaces. The reflected pulse timing from these interfaces arriving back at the head at position A would be A to B x 2, A to C x 2, etc. The timing of these returns continuously repeated and at different angles would form the basis of an electronically derived picture. An image is formed by the electronics based on the angle and timing of the returned pulses compared to the initial one that was transmitted. This contrasts with therapeutic ultrasound in that in the ideal situation no reflections would occur, but in the reality, they do. The stream of therapeutic ultrasound pulses entering and being reflected off a foetus may cause hyperaemia in the foetus that may not be beneficial. This condition along with the unnatural stimulation of stem cells, as discussed earlier, may cause growth abnormalities. Other areas where the use of therapeutic ultrasound may cause problems is over and around tumour sites. Hyperaemia normally causes a beneficial response, but in this case, it may have other effects. It could increase the temperature of the tumour itself, that in turn increases its metabolism and growth. Add to this the possibility of metastasising caused by the physical vibrations.

The same logic contraindicating therapeutic ultrasound is in any condition where a rise in temperature is to be avoided. Typical of these is where there are acute infections as contraindicated with certain other electrotherapies previously mentioned. The known and proven effect of shortwave ultrasound applied to any tissue is thermal. Applying around an infected area would cause an increase in blood flow as temperature around the infection is added to. This may efficiently spread the infection beyond the original infected area. General contraindications discussed above, and others are listed below:

1. Active bone growth plates
2. Acute infections
3. Exposed neural tissue
4. If the patient is pregnant
5. Malignant or cancerous tissue
6. On or near the eye
7. Recent history of venous thrombosis
8. Risk of haemorrhage
9. Suspicion of a bone fracture
10. Severely ischaemic tissue
11. Use in the region of sex organs (the gonads)
12. Young animals or children

Further reasoning for the above contraindications are given in turn as follows:

1. Active bone plates continue to be contraindicated for some time into early adulthood. Only when fully fused, as shown on radiographs, could ultrasound therapy be safely applied. Research has shown that Increases in the thickness of the plate caused by ultrasound could cause a difference in length of long bones thereby causing possible future problems associated with gait abnormalities.

2. Acute infections as discussed above may be made worse by the heating effect to adjacent uninfected tissue. The resulting blood vessel dilation response to increased temperature could quickly spread the infection.

3. Exposed neural tissue would occur with new injuries. Lesions naturally have severed nerves that play a part in the healing process. If such nerves are afferent types A and C proprioceptor nerves, then ultrasound stimulation may further cause both acute and chronic pain responses.

4. Pregnancy, the difference between imaging ultrasound and therapeutic was discussed earlier in this chapter. Cavitation is not likely to occur with imaging methods but could with short wave if applied close to the uterus. Direct damage to developing foeti is possible. Also, unnaturally temperature rises, such as hyperaemia, may alter foetal cellular metabolism.

5. Malignant tumours by their very nature can metastasise. Applying any stimulus near or into a tumour site could exacerbate the process.

6. Eyes are very sensitive areas of the body. The nature of their construction contains semi-liquids as in the aqueous and vitreous humours. The translucency of these liquids is essential for clear vision. Ultrasound entering the eye may cause opaqueness within the liquids leading to cataracts and foggy vision. Also, the rods and cones light receptor cells may be directly affected or damaged leading to blindness.

7. Thrombosis, deep vein thrombosis is mainly caused by blood clot formation in deep veins that are mainly found in the legs and pelvic regions. Some or part of these clots may break free and lodge within the lung. Applying ultrasound to areas where possible clot formations occur, usually in the upper limb, may cause breakdown of any clots into smaller ones that may go on to cause causing pulmonary embolisms.

8. Risk of haemorrhage is particularly contraindicated. There are many different types of haemorrhage from those within the brain associated with strokes such as subarachnoid haemorrhage to those from ruptured blood vessels elsewhere within the body. The use of ultrasound is generally contraindicated around the head but elsewhere, where swelling from injury is present, there is a need to find out if the swelling is a fluid reaction or caused by a bleed. The most obvious of these is the haematoma resulting from a fracture, See item 9 below. As with other conditions, heating effect would cause vascular dilation and if in the region of a haemorrhage would exacerbate the condition.

9. Possible bone fractures are where stress or semi-fractures occur especially in long bones. Healing process should follow the standard pattern of bleeding, oedema and callus formation. Any fracture is painful due to the high number of pain nociceptors found in the periosteum. The use of ultrasound may increase pain sensations and cause extra unnecessary bleeding.

10. Severely ischaemic tissue: Problematic blood vessels caused by blockages or narrowing can lead to lack of blood and oxygen in tissue. Normal cellular metabolism is reduced or halted, and this can lead, in the more extreme cases, to tissue death or simply cause the tissue to severely dysfunction. The heating effect associated with short wave ultrasound would not necessarily cause vasodilation or increased metabolism in

ischaemic tissue since the prime cause of the narrowing or blockages may be due to other factors. However, ultrasound is contraindicated as it is largely unknown and unresearched for this condition.

11. Use in the region of sex organs (the gonads) could create problems as they are temperature sensitive. Gonad is the name given to ovaries in females and testes in males. Because of their external location in males, testes are more susceptible to injury and damage than female ovaries. Production of sperm and hormones can be affected if ideal conditions of temperature, pressure and general environment are not maintained. Whilst the same considerations should apply to ultrasound around ovaries, and, like inhibited spermatozoa production, gamete production may be also adversely affected. Using on testes may also illicit a pain response as well as a more concentrated increase in temperature which would be likely to occur in such a confined space.

12. Young animals or children are particularly susceptible to changes caused by ultrasound applied around growth plates. An example has already been discussed in item 1 of this list and earlier in this chapter from a research project where a 25% increase across the gap was caused with very little stimulation from shortwave ultrasound. It follows that anywhere on developing young animals or children overstimulation may occur leading to unnatural or disproportionate growth in those areas of the body. Ultrasound is therefore contraindicated for the young.

Much of the research on shortwave ultrasound has been around joint problems, notably osteoarthritis and these have proven very positive. Tascioglu [24] (2010) in The *Journal of International Medical Research* reports a Turkish University study using shortwave ultrasound on human patients knee osteoarthritic problems that interestingly not only compared the results from

1MHz application at 2Watts/cm^2 applied constantly but also using a pulsed setting. WOMAC [27] (Western Ontario and McMaster Universities osteoarthritis index 1982) scoring methods showed significantly higher scores than placebo patients. The pulse setting appeared to be more effective than the constant setting. My own assessment of this would be that allowing a short interval that interrupts the constant stream of ultrasound energy inhibits saturation and allows assimilation of the energy more efficiently. This is typical of some other electrotherapies such as pulsed magnetic therapy.

General Discussion

Shortwave ultrasound by its very nature is the high energy, low penetration, superficially effective treatment for a variety of conditions. The most obvious beneficial effect is thermal. Others are stimulation and helping to optimise certain conditions to heal where other factors may be slowing the process. As discussed in this chapter, it is not an 'off-the-shelf' modality for the professional therapist that may be bought and applied without training and good knowledge of its application and contraindications.

Chapter Six

Longwave Ultrasound

Much of the previous chapter has been a discussion on short wave ultrasound. Some general comparisons identifying the differences between longwave and shortwave therapy were discussed, also the safety aspects of longwave suggest that it is possible safer to apply due to the very much lower probability of unstable cavitation developing. With this lower frequency comes the ability to penetrate deeper into tissue. However, research on longwave ultrasound is very sparse and inconclusive at this time although some positive findings have been included in this dedicated chapter.

Attenuation can be described as a comparison between the amount of energy applied in comparison to the amount measured at certain depths into tissue at 1cm intervals. This, like audible sound, is measured in decibels. Since the decibel is a logarithmic scale of sound pressure 0dB (a positive value) to over 120dB (threshold of pain) this represents the pressure difference, as discussed in chapter 2, of 1,000,000,000. Put simply for every 10 decibel (dB) increase in sound pressure, the sound intensity is ten times as loud. 30dB would be 1000 times and 40db 10000, and so on. Some sources put the threshold of pain at 130dB which is 10 times louder than that.

The above discussion may be considered academic, but the principles of measuring pressure differentials remains the same with all energy gains and losses. With ultrasound and any other form of energy transfer, decibel scales are used. The use of dead animal tissue, such as pork has allowed comparative measurements through purely soft tissue or a mixture of soft and hard tissue such as through the ribcage. An original paper from *Circulation*, the journal of the American Heart Association [1] reports how attenuation measurements were made by placing two types of transducers in the tissue. Hydrophones and thermocoupled sensors like our own shortwave ultrasound experiment. Hydrophones measured the actual ultrasound energy and the thermo-couples measured the temperature change caused by the energy absorption into the tissue.

A standard measurement that translates to an attenuation factor of 50% is 3dB. It was found that attenuation of 40KHz longwave was reduced by 3dB per cm. This was measured through the ribcage and is attributed to a mixture of hard and soft tissue being more absorbent and scattering than soft tissue alone. However, very little attenuation occurs when passing purely through soft tissue. This would mean that there is little absorption and energy dispersion and very much longer times of application would be required to treat superficial areas to achieve the same energy density as shortwave ultrasound. However, it does mean that deeper tissue may be reached than with shortwave ultrasound.

Longwave ultrasound, like all energy transfers used in therapy, is affected by the ability of the medium to absorb the available energy that in turn relates proportionately to the scattering of the energy. This means that if various conditions to be targeted require higher amounts of energy to be effective, then transmission through any medium such as soft tissue would require a focussed beam to arrive at target tissue relatively intact. It is virtually impossible to keep the cohesiveness of any ultrasound beam temporally together through a soft but still relatively dense medium such as body tissue. Even a laser beam loses temporal cohesion when passing through air. This can be demonstrated by shining a laser pen across a room at a wall. The very narrow beam that leaves the pen is slightly dispersed by air molecules forming a broader spot on the wall surface. All low sound frequencies naturally widely disperse, and long-wave ultrasound is no exception. The nature of the relatively high longwave ultrasound frequency used would be, to some extent, directable from the head, a wide dispersion would naturally begin to occur as soon as it enters tissue. This may be overcome by:

1. Selecting equipment with a concave applicator head
2. Using higher power settings
3. Targeting through intervening soft tissue

Discussing these in turn:

1. The availability of a focussing head for longwave applicators are, at the time of writing, not yet available. Most long-wave heads that I have seen are domed, suggesting a wide dispersion from the start.
2. The use of higher power settings is a two-edged sword in that the most energetic part of the ultrasound energy is at the skin surface.
3. Although longwave energy transmits well through tissue, this wide dispersion would affect other structures not necessarily targeted. This may not be a bad thing as there is little evidence of any detrimental effect found in research.

The other aspect is the equipment itself. Since therapists often require that equipment be portable, when offering a peripatetic service, then available battery power and duration needs to be a factor considered before treatment. Most portable equipment utilises sealed 12Volt lead-acid batteries that can deliver a high current. If the rating of the battery is a standard 1.3 Amps per hour, then a 4watt/cm^2 head covering 4 cm^2 head would require 16 Watts of energy. Since Power in Watts = Current in Amps x Voltage (P = I x V), then I= P/V = 16/12 = 1.33Amps. This means that on full power a fully charged battery would theoretically last just 1 hour before requiring recharging. Some applicators are larger than 4 cm^2 and power settings are also higher. These problems can be overcome by using larger batteries but come with a proportionate increase in weight and time to recharge. Bearing in mind these factors for portable use, planning is required to include considering the number of patients to be treated, duration of each treatment, possibility of charging, say from a car auxiliary socket whilst in transit, the possibility of carrying a spare fully charged battery that can quickly and easily be fitted as needed and the size of the head, if interchangeable.

Targeting specific conditions and areas through tissue, one condition suggested in various sources that could benefit from longwave ultrasound is a sprained ankle. In 1996 Bradnock[4] carried out comparative research between longwave and shortwave ultrasound on sprained ankles. This research was placebo driven with active and sham applications at frequencies of 45KHz and 3 MHz, respectively. The 'Gait-way' system of assessment found that the patient's gait was statistically improved immediately after treatment using longwave ultrasound in comparison with shortwave. Gait-way method of assessment was developed by the University of Salford mainly on paediatric patients. This research would suggest that the high energy levels found in shortwave ultrasound are not an important factor. I would further suggest that, at these lower longwave frequencies, the idea of 'micro-massage' having a therapeutic internal effect may be a reality causing some pain reduction leading to an improved gait.

Chapter Seven

SHOCKWAVE THERAPY

Direct contact therapies have necessarily to include ones that are likely to be encountered but not therapeutic in the normal recovery sense. Shockwave units are in more widespread use by veterinary practices and knowledge of them is essential for therapists to both understand the reason for their use and their likely effects. Shockwave is classed as a therapy but is used to treat conditions in an unusual way from the other electrotherapies being discussed in this book and in the two previous ones in the series. Its use is generally limited to use by veterinary surgeon, due to the need to sedate or anaesthetise animals to be treated. Post-treatment cases may well require the services of a physiotherapist and therefore knowledge of its design, use and likely effects is essential.

In the previous chapter the energy aspect of ultrasound therapy was discussed but shockwave, another type of direct contact therapy, needs to be included. It uses high energetic mechanical pressure pulses targeted directly at specific injuries within tissue. Shockwave's full title is Extracorporeal Shock Wave Therapy (ESWT). The term 'extracorporeal' meaning outside of the body could be used with any of the other ultrasound therapies but is really only ever applied to Shockwave. ESWT is not ultrasound in the context of this section of the book, but it is frequently found in veterinary practices and has some similarities with longwave ultrasound therapy. Usually, shockwave pulses are emitted from the applicator varying from a single pulse up to 2000Hz. They are of extremely high intensity. Shockwave treatments are exactly as the title suggests in that they apply shocks to tissue. This form of electrotherapy is from a transducer that provides a very high intensity mechanical pressure impact, sometimes in a short repetitive chain or 'bursts' of up to 2000 or more pulses targeting problem areas. Some of the original theories behind this type of therapy is that it can be applied to old unresolved injuries to 'reboot' the natural healing process particularly with orthopaedic problems such as non-union fractures. However, its historical use has been to resolve renal problems (lithotripsy) in human patients, typically kidney stones (urinary calculosis) or other areas where stones can form, such as gall bladder, liver and pancreas. These have been successfully treated by it causing the stones to shatter and thereby allowing them to dissolve or pass more easily without invasive surgery.

The basis of shockwave development arose in Germany in 1962. The defence ministry investigated the effect of shock waves on tissue. This resulted in the development of the 'Lithotripter' by the University of Munich for renal use. The first application took place in 1980 and by 1984 it was given approval by the Drug Enforcement Administration (DEA) in the United States.

With the use on human patients the list of potential problems that could be treated by shockwave is extensive. Many manufacturers extol the efficacy of their product with many examples for its application. These range in human treatments from painful foot conditions such as:

- Plantar fasciitis/heel-pain
- Achilles Tendinopathy
- Patella Tendinopathy
- Adductor Tendinopathy
- Hamstring Tendinopathy
- Glute Tendinopathy/Greater Trochanteric Pain Syndrome
- De Quervains Tenosynovitis
- Tennis Elbow
- Golfers Elbow
- Shoulder/Rotator Cuff Tendinopathies including Calcific Tendinitis

There are several designs of applicators, allowing either radial or a single point concentration of energy. They can be a concave reflective type that focuses the shock wave on to a specific point, or some wide-beam convex radial applicators covering a larger area. Others include multiple devices that increase focus and energy by simultaneous application from different angles all focussed on one point.

A paper by Schmitz [22] (2015), states in the research section that there is no scientific evidence in favour of focussed shock wave or of radial shockwave. The basis of this is that the energy of the shockwave pulses is a minor consideration given the fact that energy originating from a radial device will be absorbed and diminish very quickly once in tissue. However, since it is of much higher intensity and lower frequency than ultrasound therapies the intensity of the pulses are still high enough to cause the desired effects deeper into tissue.

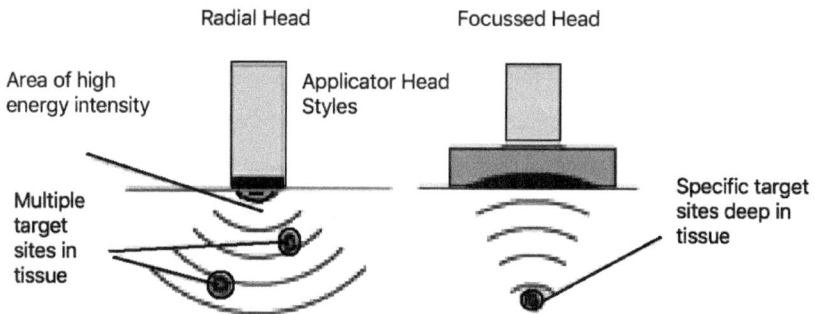

Figure 15. Stylised representations of radial and focussed shockwave applicators

Shock waves are generated by several different means, Piezo-electric, electromagnetic and oil sparked. Piezoelectric ones share a common use of a property of quartz with therapeutic ultrasound. In the case of shock wave a very large but short duration electric pulse is applied across a crystal causing it to instantly change shape. This deformation is transmitted to the applicator head to be further transmitted as a high-pressure mechanical shock wave into tissue. The crystal almost instantly regains its natural state until the next pulse comes along. These types are ideal for rapid chains of pulses used in some applications. Electromagnetic devices are akin to a loudspeaker. A circular magnet is accelerated through the centre of coil of wire due to the attraction caused by the coil being quickly energised. The rapid movement of the magnet then hits a stop sending a shock wave though it that is again transmitted to tissue. This type has frequency limitations but can be very energetic. The oil spark generator develops the pressure wave by rapid expansion of heat generated between two electrodes strategically positioned in an oil chamber. A high-voltage pulse causes an electric arc discharge between the electrodes. The almost instantaneous rise to a very high temperature vaporises the oil around the electrodes and this causes a rapid expansion pressure wave that can be focused forward by design of the applicator head. The oil cools the area of the electrodes very quickly such that the process can be quickly repeated to deliver multiple mechanical shocks. This method could be described as electro-hydraulic in its action.

Early examples of shockwave-type devices were used in research based around investigating the healing state of long-bone fractures in humans. Somewhat primitive methods were employed to initiate a transverse acceleration along the bone to the fracture site. The changes in this acceleration 'signal' would then be analysed proximally and then distally to the fracture using Fourier analysis to note successive changes as the healing phase of the fracture progressed. Various methods were employed including firing an airgun pellet aimed safely and carefully at a small plate over the tibial tuberosity of the fractured tibia. This caused a resulting transverse shock-wave to be transmitted down the bone. Others dropped ball bearings of a specific weight from a predetermined height to achieve a similar shock-wave. Both could quickly result in pain if applied too often. My own research developed a lighter weight but fast pulsing impactor that had much less discomfort for the patient but still provided the relevant data. It was named by the department's professor as the 'Salford Impactor'. The above research example is included to give an illustration in practice as to exactly what a shockwave acceleration is. It is unlikely that shockwave applicators used in this context would be encountered by therapist and no long term after-effects would be likely to need treatment.

Treatment regimes

In discussing shockwave therapy with veterinary surgeons, it was a surprise to find that it was very frequently used as a general treatment. In the context of unresolved fractures, shockwave should not be applied as a repeated therapy, as once the fracture site is initialised and in a bleeding phase, normal healing processes should follow. Repeated use of shockwave could inhibit the repair processes. However, there may be other factors that cause a delay in the healing that are believed to be neurological. If the nerves serving the fracture site or indeed around it are damaged, research by Becker [2] (1985) suggests that the injury may be delayed in being resolved. This healing process is slowed down or halted until the nerve fibres reconnect. This is a theory that is applied to fracture healing where, in humans, delayed or non-union occurs in up to 20% of damaged long bones. Regular application of shockwave therapy to these fractures may cause repeated initialisation and further damage to the nerves and may cause further delay. It may also cause stress fractures in the region of the initial injury if applied too often.

Further recommendations from the *British Medical Bulletin* [22] (2015) in the PEDro database suggested that the ideal was weekly treatments set at 2000 pulses per second at the highest energy level tolerable by the patient.

Because shockwave is usually applied to sedated animals, it may be out of the range of treatments usually encountered by the therapist but recovery regimes treatments for dealing with the aftermath may well need to be met. Typical responses may be swelling as haematomas could result along with chronic pain developing. Shock wave is a stimulation to trigger healing. As mentioned before, no therapy can heal or increase the rate of healing.

The conditions that manufacturers claim to be suitable for shockwave treatments are extensive. Claims of a 65% to 85% success rate given by some research sources and clinics should perhaps be weighed against the fact that many conditions resolve themselves naturally and it has to be assumed that the above figures were obtained from troublesome cases where natural processes were absent. Both medical and veterinary sources suggest that the 70% figure is about the rate for non-surgical non-diseased or infected conditions that go through an acute stage followed by a chronic stage to naturally healing. It may be that certain of these conditions, where natural healing is delayed, will be 'kick-started' by shock wave applications. Other sources suggest that the following list of conditions are suitable for ESWT on animals and have a similarity to the human treatment list mention earlier in this chapter.

Tendon problems seem the ideal areas for treatment in both human and animal patients. With animal treatments, feedback from veterinary physiotherapists who also are employed in veterinary practices, suggest that horses will tolerate shockwave treatment. Smaller animals are less well able to be treated unless fully anaesthesised. The subject and use of shockwave therapy had initially a mixed reception. With many vets now using the equipment along with others that are perhaps a little more sceptical, its acceptance may well increase with time as research and case histories are reported.

Shockwave research

Interesting reading on shockwave research can be found in an article labelled: 'Efficiency and safety of extracorporeal conditions: a systematic review on studies listed on PEDro database' by Schmitz [21](2015) This paper can be easily found on the internet and is useful for those wishing to learn more about its efficacy in resolving certain conditions based on a large number listed in the PEDro database. A review summarised from the discussions found within this document suggests the following:

1. The effectiveness of shockwave is suggested from cumulative data to be around 85.5%. A discussion around these values when applied to orthopaedics was found earlier in this chapter.

2. For various treatments using this modality, many case studies suggest that it is safe to use with no reports of any adverse effects. This conclusion came about from the many random controlled trials (RCTs).

3. A possible negative result is where shockwave is applied to animals where localised anaesthesia is given.

Chapter Eight

DIRECT ELECTRICAL STIMULATION THERAPIES

Muscle Stimulators

These types of direct stimulators cause muscles to contract or twitch by being applied at the skin surface along the line of a target muscle group. Muscle stimulators can be characterised by high and low voltage levels along with pulsing rates. High-voltage stimulators are sometimes referred to as 'Faradic' and can be used to help increase muscle mass by causing controlled contractions. Others can use much lower voltages applied in similar ways to simply condition muscles where injury has occurred. This chapter mainly deals with the high-voltage types to give understanding of the processes involved before finally considering lower-voltage stimulation.

To understand how they achieve their effect, there is a need to look at how muscles contract naturally from signals arising in the brain to enable a contraction of a specific group of muscles. Voltages above 50 Volts can be considered potentially lethal to both humans and animals; understanding both the effect and nature of how such high voltages can be safely applied is essential for any therapists wishing to use this modality. This chapter aims to achieve this by looking at simple electrical principles alongside of the more complicated electrochemical processes involved in the body.

The term voltage can be described as the electrical pressure or charge that propels electrons between negative and positive electrical sources. The level of charge is called the potential difference between a negative source with an abundance of electrons and a positive one that lacks electrons. If a material capable of conducting current is linked between them, negatively charged electrons will form a current flowing from the negative to the positive connections. This is electron current flow. Conventional current flow describes it as flowing from positive to negative. This comes from the 1900s before the discovery of electrons but is still called conventional current flow and used in circuit dynamics to this day. The amount of current flow is measured in amperes (I) and is limited by the resistance offered by the conducting material (R). This resistance has a value and is measured in ohms. The simple relationship is V = I x R. In this section of the book voltages discussed range voltages up to, and in excess o,f 100 Volts, used in direct muscle stimulation.

The term potential difference is also applied to the seemingly very low charge, found across the membrane of cells, that attracts selective positively charged particles to the negatively charged interior of the cell through selective membrane channels. These are nutrients such as sodium (Na^-) that are negatively charged. These are called cations. Conversely charged molecules such as potassium (P^+) are call anions and are attracted out of the cell. Both the inflow and outflow are through special channels in the membrane. The flow of these charged molecules is not generally described as a current in the same sense as that flowing along a wire and is rarely if ever measured in amperes. However, the principles are the same. As with any electrotherapy, training is essential in use of the modality not only to achieve maximum benefit but for safe application. Muscle (faradic) stimulation operates with high voltages and so, as with any electrical stimulation therapies, safety for both patient and therapist can be compromised if not applied correctly.

Conscious control to make muscles contract requires the brain to generates a series of action potentials and send them down to the muscle via efferent myelinated alpha type nerves of the central nervous system, followed by similar nerves of the peripheral nervous system. The nerve fibres are known as axons and are in the alpha type 1 grouping. These action potentials are produced in the brain by decision making neurons in the motor cortex and fed via a complex of dendrites to a motor neuron. Once certain conditions are met by a weighted system of inputs, the electric potential at its descending axon hillock (see figure 16) is caused to exceed a certain threshold. An avalanche effect occurs when this threshold is exceeded, rapidly opening and attracting sodium through selective axon membrane channels. These are then opened sequentially by the change in membrane potential voltage all along the membrane of the axon.

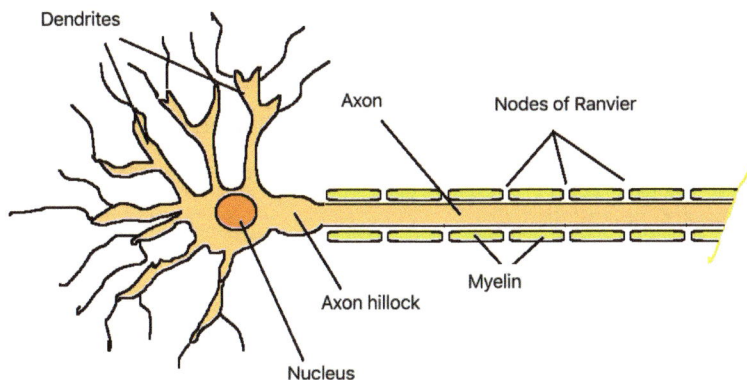

Figure 16. Neuron and axon formation

This can be likened to a 'Mexican wave'. The axon membrane at its resting potential is polarised, electrically sitting at around the minus (-) 70mV level (negative on the inside, positive on the outer). The inflow of sodium from the interstitial fluid changes this potential to around plus (+) 30mV as the 360^0 'Mexican wave' of the action potential passes. The potential eventually returns to its -70mV resting voltage after briefly reaching a 'hyperpolarised' level of around -90mV until the next action potential comes along.

Figure 17 below is an illustration of the process where the action potential travelling from right to left changes the voltage gradient across the axon membrane. The membrane is surrounded by glial cells referred to as myelin. These are cells that wrap around the axon forming a myelin sheath insulative barrier to the outside tissue and interstitial fluid. The myelin has some gaps between one another although some physical contact is maintained. These gaps are access points for the inflow of sodium and are called 'Nodes of Ranvier'. As the action potential passes it slightly affects the next Node of Ranvier area, preconditioning sodium channels and speeding up the inflow of sodium. This has the effect of accelerating the transit of action potentials along the axon. This speeding up is called 'saltatory' conduction where saltatory means to leap. Excess sodium flows out of the axon again through selective channels attracted by the temporary imbalance and depletion of sodium ions caused in the area by passing action potentials.

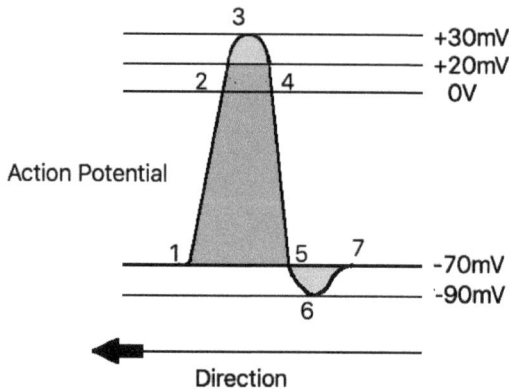

Figure 17. Typical action potential

The numbers above in the above diagram indicate:

1. Resting potential (-70mV)
2. Zero-volt level increasing
3. Peak level (+30mV)
4. Zero-volt level decreasing
5. Passing through resting potential (-70mV)
6. Hyperpolarising level (-90mV)
7. Return to resting potential (-70mV)

Between 4 and 5 would be the sodium outflow from the axon.

The time taken from the start of the action potential to it restoring the resting -70V potential is call the 'absolute refractory time'. Subsequent action potentials cannot impinge on this, thus setting the highest repetition rates allowed for a particular fibre that may be at many thousands per second. The overall potential gradient in the 70mV to 130mV range that is measured across the membranes, represents about 3,000,000 Volts per metre. This is due to the thickness of the membrane being about 7 to 9 nm (nanometres, one nm being one thousand millionth of a metre). See in references that some suggest as low as 3nm thickness.

As the voltage across the membrane passes through zero into the positive level, this causes selective sodium channels to start to open allowing an inflow of sodium into the axon as discussed above. However, the neurons not only generate axon potentials but also manufacture neurotransmitters such as acetylcholine (ACh). These are transferred in vesicles through microtubules within and along the length of the axon through a migratory system called fast axonal transport or drift.

ACh is required to transmit the action potential across chemical synapses and at the neuromuscular junction called the motor endplate. The vesicles are released into a synaptic cleft separating the presynaptic neuron and the motor endplate. This is caused by the action potential opening voltage- gated channels in the presynaptic membrane. The ACh is released into and then crosses the cleft and is attracted to bind to ACh receptors on the postsynaptic neuron and on the very much larger area of receptors on the neuromuscular junction. This again generates a wider action potential along the length of the junction that radiates across the sarcolemma and throughout the muscle via t-tubules conduits. This is said to polarise the muscle. Momentary polarisation causes voltage sensitive proteins in calcium channels within the membrane of the sarcoplasmic reticulum to open. Calcium released through the sarcoplasmic reticulum channels then quickly permeates into the muscle fibres called sarcomeres. At this point it would be simple to say that the net effect of this polarising voltage is to cause a contraction of the sarcomere, but for those who wish to understand fully the process, the next couple of paragraphs and diagrams may provide some explanation.

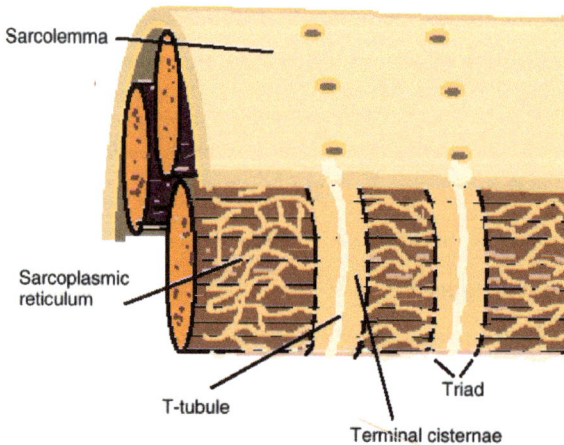

Figure 18. Action potential conduits into muscle

A sarcomere is a contractile basic muscle unit found in striated skeletal and cardiac muscles. It is comprised of two basic components, thin and thick filaments, see figure 20 below.

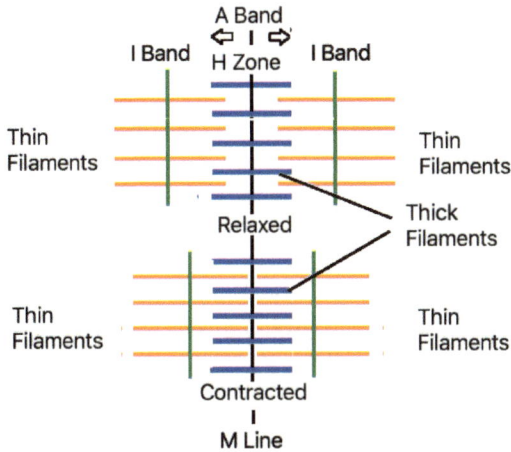

Figure 19. Representation of striated muscle structure

The thick and thin filaments are myosin and actin strands, respectively. Adenosine triphosphate (ATP) is attached to the myosin thick filaments and the actin thin filaments have binding sites and troponin cross bridges. When calcium is released from the sarcoplasmic reticulum following muscle polarisation, tropomyosin covering the binding sites, is caused to change shape exposing them. Cross bridges then link the ATP to the binding sites and in the process the ATP loses a phosphate molecule to become ADP (adenosine diphosphate) changing its shape. This change of shape is the power stroke that causes the actin myosin filaments to slide together momentarily before releasing the cross bridges. This is repeated throughout the muscle many millions of times causing the muscle to shorten. It does not return to its pre-contracted shape by itself but is relaxed and an antagonist muscle operates to extend the muscle back to its normal uncontracted length. For readers wishing to study this process deeper there are some good internet sites demonstrating the process of muscle contractions with animations.

To cause muscles to contract, a chain of action potentials is sent by the brain. This keeps the sarcomere shortened and engages other sarcomeres to increase the strength and amount of the overall contraction. A single action potential would probably just result in almost undiscernible twitch of the muscle. With electric current stimulation we try to mimic the chain of pulses with an electrical potential capable of causing the release of calcium into the sarcomere over a wide range within the body of the muscle. Where a potential difference, e.g. voltage (potential difference), is applied across any two points of the body, a current is established between them. Depending on where the contacts are made this can be either dangerous or beneficial. The danger comes from voltage level applied. It is known that if applied incorrectly a current of far less than 1 milliamp can be fatal. It may also be disruptive to the heart's rhythm if applied close to it.

Taking resistance measurements across any two points of the human body yields various dry skin values of around 800,000 ohms (Ω). As current (I) = Voltage (V) divided by resistance, if 50 volts is applied across these two points then current flowing (I), equals 50/800,000 = 5/80,000 or 0.0625 milliamps). This low current value may be increased if the contact point of the electric source is wet or dampened. Electrolytes within tissue may offer a much lower resistance once the surface resistance is overcome. Fifty volts and above could therefore cause a potentially increasing lethal level of current to flow. Faradic stimulators work at voltages of up to 220 Volts but are applied in such a way that processes the voltage and mitigates the lethal nature of such a high potential.

The 800,000Ω value mentioned earlier arises by measuring at the surface on relatively dry human skin. If the skin is damp due to being in contact with either water or sweat, then this lowers the observed resistance by around 50%. Gel electrical connection pads or the use of an electrically conductive gel where rubberised pads are used, provide a connection that allows current to enter tissue more easily. Subcutaneous fats and muscle comprised mainly of water along with electrolytes provide a lowered resistance forming a direct pathway between the two electrical connections from the equipment. This effectively means that other nearby structures that may offer an alternative pathway, such as metal plates joining fracture segments, should not compromise the treatment by diverting away from this direct pathway. This is provided that the distance between the two pads, forming the circuit, is shorter in length.

There are five aspects to be considered when faradic stimulation is to be applied:

1. Suitability of both the patient and condition to be treated
2. The area to be targeted
3. The voltage as just mentioned above
4. The rate of pulses applied
5. Duration of each treatment.

1. The suitability of the patient for faradic treatment is best arrived at by discussions with a veterinary surgeon or doctor referring the case forward. Conditions such as epilepsy and cardiac failure might be contraindicated if in the patient's medical history. Infected areas may also be considered problematic due to increases in temperature if close to the muscles needing stimulation.
2. Surface anatomy knowledge is important to enable specific muscle groups to be targeted. Application should always be along the muscles and positioned in such a way that only the agonist is caused to twitch or momentarily contract.

3. All muscle stimulators should have variable output controls affecting both the frequency of the pulses and the output intensity. Treatments should always start with the output level set to a low level and slowly increased. If distress is caused, then the treatment should cease immediately.

4. To elicit an initial twitch, the frequency of the pulses should also be set very low, perhaps to just one pulse per second. Coupled with the output level, this should remain low and slowly increased until a twitch of the muscle is observed. Provided the patient does not display any form of distress, then once this initial twitch level has been achieved, the frequency may be increased in small steps, but carefully observing the patient's reaction.

5. Timing is important because, as was observed with paraplegic patients discussed later in this chapter, atrophied muscles quickly fatigue. Setting a specific time of application may well depend upon the severity of the initial injury causing the problem. A few minutes of application would probably be a good start until evidence of increased muscle mass and a good contraction reaction is established.

A mitigating factor reducing the possibility of high voltages directly causing damage is achieved by the voltage pulses being of very short duration and by the careful placement of the electrodes. This is so that electric current flow is limited to the target area only. Also, it is possible to cause a burn at the sites of the applicator pads if voltage levels are set too high and applied for too long. Electric current flow established between two connecting pads will always take the easiest and shortest path of least resistance. This means that if applied along a specific muscle group the current will largely remain confined to flowing along that set of muscles, leaving other adjacent structures largely unaffected. See Figure 20 below:

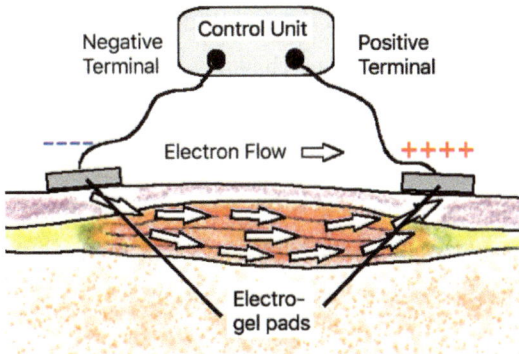

Figure. 20. Electron current flow along and through a muscle.

The above diagram shows a stylised muscle with electrodes (connecting pads) attached at the skin surface. The potentials being applied are represented by the minus and plus signs above them. The current flow is likely to take a broader path through the muscle than shown and is dependent upon the level of the potential difference between the pads.

As a pulse of current passes through the muscle it appears to have the same effect as an action potential generated post-synapse at the neuromuscular junction. This voltage change is radiated throughout the muscle by t-tubules conduits causing calcium-gated channels to open flooding the sarcomere with calcium. Externally applied voltages would not follow a specific t-tubule route throughout the muscle but may effectively saturate the whole body of the muscle forcing membrane potential changes and affecting voltage controlled gated calcium channels. This would result in them opening, thus mimicking action potentials initiated naturally. Although potentials above 50 Volts are commonly used to stimulate, causing some contraction in skeletal muscles, the use of very much lower low-voltage stimulators can be used to some effect.

In the case of muscles that are in the chronic stage of recovery, where loading and function is severely restricted, the use of low-voltage pulsing devices may begin to slightly open the calcium channels in the sarcoplasmic reticulum allowing a small amount of calcium into the sarcomere. This will elicit a small series of micro-twitches from them. These are insufficient to cause any meaningful contraction of the muscle but will allow some conditioning whilst the muscle is necessarily inactive. This effect can be safely demonstrated by attaching two electro-pads along the adductor muscles of the lower arm. With the low-voltage equipment set to a base frequency of 50Hz pulsing at around 5 to ten times per second, a small sensation will be felt in the muscle at voltages between 6 to 12 Volts. This is the muscle being caused to twitch by very few of the sarcomeres being engaged.

The suitability of the patient for direct stimulation treatment covers a wide spectrum for use both with humans and animals. The most successful use of faradic stimulation, in my experience, was in human use. It was used to increase the mass and restore some function of hypo-trophic (atrophied) muscles in the lower limbs of paraplegic patients. This research was carried out by the Department of Orthopaedic Mechanics from the University of Salford in the early 1990s. This research was associated with Manchester University's School of Medicine at the clinical sciences department of Hope Hospital and had patients with spinal lesions arising from various accidents. Typical of these were mainly young males from accidents with motorcycles. They were deemed to be suitable candidates because their overall fitness was good despite the obvious physical limitations. Over a period, the patient's legs were stimulated by targeting muscle groups that would initiate a kick reaction. Initially the patients were suspended by being sat on a bicycle-like device with the stimulator pads attached over the soleus and gastrocnemius muscles with the legs hanging freely. These muscle groups were stimulated sequentially between left and right. In the initial phase of treatment virtually no response was noted from the long unused muscles. As the stimulation sessions continued over weeks and months, the muscle groups began to contract and eventually the muscle caused the legs to swing below the knee. A rapid growth was also noted in the muscle mass.

The whole purpose of this research was to see if sufficient reactivation build-up and strengthening of the muscle could lead to the subjects being able to support themselves and, with electro-stimulative assistance, be able to be mobilised with the aid of reciprocating gate arthrosis devices. The most successful subject gained sufficient muscle build up and strength to be able to walk through service tunnel of the channel tunnel at speeds matching his able-bodied supporters. This event was organised as fundraiser.

The above example was carried out with a team of doctors and medical scientists in support. However, it is unlikely in veterinary application that paraplegic animals would be physically or psychologically able to be treated in the way described above but the example is included to show just what faradic stimulation can achieve. The most obvious type of injury where muscle stimulation would be useful with animals is in the recovery stage of serious injuries where muscles have necessarily been immobilised. This is where surgery has taken place as in the pinning or plating of fractures. Over the recovery phase, muscle will lose some mass and may be aided when recovery permit, to regain mass, strength and function.

Pulse waveforms were monophasic which simply means they were only pulsed positively, see figure 21 below. The duration of each pulse would be very short and allow for a quick decay. Timing between each pulse could be varied but set at around 25 per second would achieve a muscle contraction. This should not be applied as a constant stream but interrupted to avoid overstressing the muscle and potential heating at the contact points.

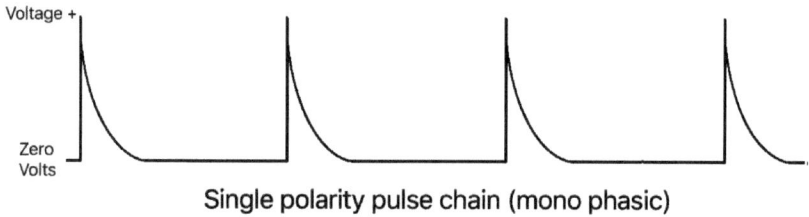

Single polarity pulse chain (mono phasic)

Figure. 21. Single polarity (monophasic) pulse chain

The illustration in figure 21 above illustrating part of a single polarity pulse chain, is seen with a slight exponential delay. This could be termed a 'reactive decay' and is a characteristic of all switching circuits caused in the electronics. It is overemphasised here and elongated. It should not be confused with 'H' wave delays discussed below where the decay is purposefully slowed down.

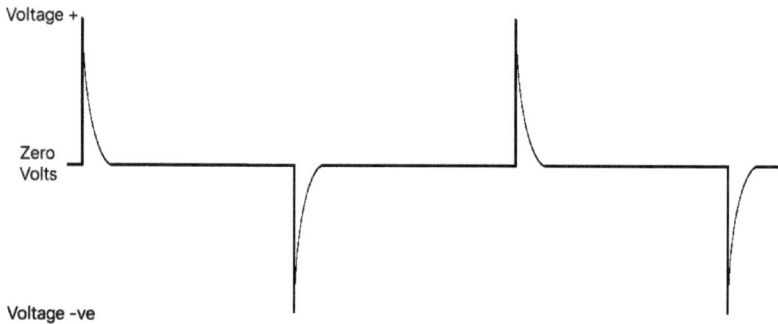

Figure 22. Dual polarity (biphasic) pulse chain

Dual polarity as shown above in figure 22 is simply a switching of the pulses applied so that the stimulating current is reversed. It applies pulses in the same way as monophasic ones in figure 21 above but effectively halves the pulse rate for each polarity. A 120 Hz chain of pulses would be divided to 60 positive and to 60 negative.

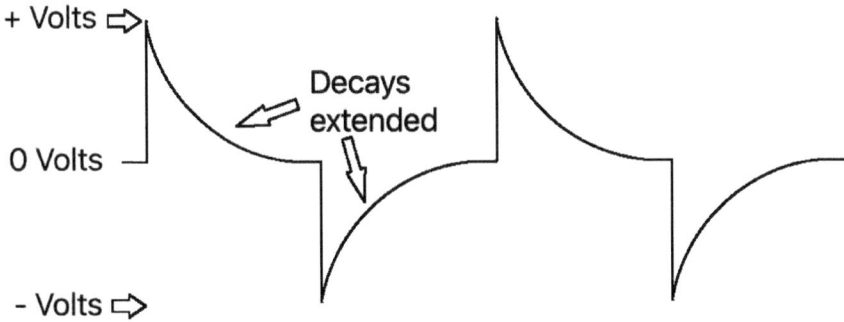

Figure 23. Bi-Phasic 'H' Wave

Figure 23 above is a biphasic waveform where the decay is purposely slowed down. This means that a positive or negative voltage is applied for longer as it decays because of the longer time to return to the zero-volt level. It is suggested that stimulating muscles to contract is more effective using this applied waveform and can be effective from just 2 pulses per second. Various manufactures market these devices to be applied both on humans and animal patients in the same way and can be used to replace TENS devices as it also suggested to have an analgesic effect. This, and the gate theory of pain, will be discussed later in chapter ten.

Discussion

The potential difference used to stimulate muscles may be at the levels discussed and radiated throughout the muscle. To achieve the same effect with muscle stimulation generally requires that the current flow established through the muscle will have this same effect on calcium channels where proteins making them up are normally electrically sensitive to the voltage gradient changes caused by the action potential. This causes these proteins to change shape opening up the channels. Forcing an unnatural current directly through the muscle may in turn have the same effect as the natural membrane potential change on the membrane channel proteins but also may cause rapid muscle fatigue to follow if overstimulated by higher voltages than necessary being applied. This may release more calcium into the sarcomere than required. The muscle will be quickly stimulated as a result and damage to the structures may occur if rapidly repeated.

Chapter Nine

MICROCURRENT THERAPY

The idea that microcurrents abound in the body is not new. As long ago in 1830, Carlos Matteuci [17] put forward the idea that lesions were electrically active. These were proven less than thirty years later by Emile Du-Bois Reymond [5] and found to be around 1 micro-Amp (one millionth of an amp) flowing across them. The question to be asked, where do these currents originate in terms of the voltages driving them? This chapter looks more in depth at the electrical nature of tissue and the theories that led to the discovery of small direct current flows that possibly form part of the feedback and stimulation mechanisms of the body. The early part of this section concentrates on the author's experience during his doctoral studies in orthopaedics and relates back to his previous writings where a common theme of both natural and induced electrostimulation became established. Microcurrent therapy may offer another solution in assisting the healing processes of the body.

In the late-1900s there were many discoveries, theories and advances in medicine. There were also some odd theories about the electrical nature of the body and its magnetism. Many of these theories came forward along with 'experts' making claims that electricity could improve and cure virtually everything from infertility to hair loss. As a great many outlandish claims by these self-proclaimed experts were made, this era became known as a 'Golden Age of Quackery'. Magnetism, also at this time, was believed by some to have a specific frequency component and unique signatures to each organ of the body. A theory that still has believers around today but understanding that magnetic fields arise from sustained directed electron flows and that free electrons are random within tissue, cancels out the idea any that magnetic field signatures from specific parts in the body exists. The idea also that any form of DC (direct current) could exist in the body was also dismissed. However, an exception to this was the 20th-century discovery of 'perineural currents'. I have discussed and theorised about these in both of my two previous books, but for the readers of this book alone, the following paragraphs gives a possible insight into them;

American orthopaedic surgeon Dr R.O. Becker carried out experiments on reptiles that had the ability to regenerate limbs, such as newts, frogs, salamanders, etc. Summarising some of his experiments, he found that if the nerves supplying the limbs were severed then regeneration or healing, or if the limb was fractured, did not take place. The two main factors for regeneration were that normocytic or 'normalised' red blood cells containing DNA were abundant and that nerves to the limbs were intact. This led to experiments as to why the nerves played an important part in bodily repair processes. 'Hall Effect' experiments were carried out in vivo on certain nerves and they were found to be conduit for minute electric currents.

The Hall Effect experiment is a system of detecting current flows by the interaction of the micromagnetic fields forming around any microcurrents, remembering that any current flow has near light speed transit of electrons. This causes micromagnetic fields to form around the current flow because they are unidirectional. With strong static magnetic fields applied across, producing an even field perpendicular to them, a small charge is caused by the flowing electrons being slightly attracted to one side of the conducting fibre. This charge is detected by small electrodes strategically placed either side of the nerve fibre. Because these currents are believed to pass along glial cells throughout the body, originating from and returning to the brain, the title 'Perineural Currents' was given to them.

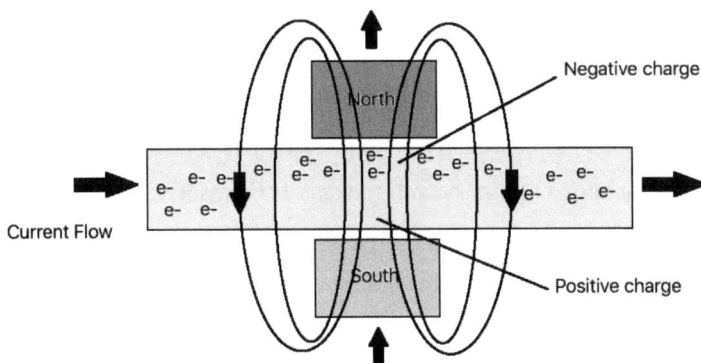

Figure 24. Hall Effect simplified diagram

The basic reason I previously put forward, based on Becker's work for the charges responsible for these currents, was that the two halves (hemispheres) of the brain differ in size. Experiments using transcranial electromagnetic stimulators and witnessed by myself on a visit with a PhD student to the University of Sheffield Department of Medical Physics in 1992, established that each side of the brain is oppositely electrically polarised. Since an electrical imbalance would be present due to the size difference of each hemisphere, then a potential (electric charge) would exist that may be felt throughout the body, this due to each half of the body being served by the opposite sides of the brain. Wherever a potential exists, then a minute current will naturally flow through tissue between charges and these could be possibly established throughout the nervous system via a conduit of lower resistance electrolytic pathways that *may* exist in glial cell cytosol. Becker labelled these currents as 'perineural currents' due to their use of myelinated cells that have some contact with each other along axons and through micro-apertures where contact is made.

'Currents of injury' refers to the existence of small currents established by charges measurable across lesions. Small nerves serving the area of the injury may have been severed and the charges arise causing 'leakage' currents through and across the lesion. Measuring these voltages may be difficult but if the resistance to current flow across the lesion is known, then this will allow the voltage to be calculated. They may form part of the body's system for stimulating the healing process until the nerves themselves heal and reconnect. The healing of bones, especially in areas abundant with still DNA bearing red blood cells in warm-blooded animals, is typical where DNA bearing 'normoblasts' are still found, these being formed within bone marrow in the process called erythropoiesis. These are known as pluripotent haemopoietic stem cells. The current across the lesion (current of injury) stimulates these pluripotent cells to be dedifferentiated to becoming structures governed by chemotactic influences of their surroundings.

The use of direct currents in medicine found some success in orthopaedics. Although there were no specific records of trials or the success rates are available, Orthopaedic surgeons, that I encountered as part of my clinical experience during my own research, would relate the fact that small currents passed through non-union fractures would often have an unexplained but positive effect. The method was to fix silver pins into the bone on either side of the fracture site, see Figure 25 below.

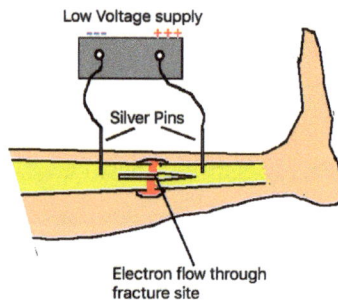

Figure 25. Direct current application to a fracture

Attaching the pins to a low-voltage source, would possibly stimulate bridging across the fracture site leading, in many cases, eventually to full union. The reason for non-union fractures was at that time unknown and the thought that nerves serving the area played an important part in the healing process was also unheard of.

Often patients would come into hospital from motorcycle accidents with bilateral fractures. One side would heal naturally but the other did not. Since the overall fitness and chemistry of these patients was identical for both injuries, the cause of non-union on one them presented a mystery. It can now be speculated that on the non-union side there may be neurological damage temporarily interrupting the nerves to the fracture site area. The theory is that If these nerves return to full function, the fracture will start to unite. If they are permanently damaged, the non-union will remain until either surgical intervention i.e. intramedullary pinning or electrostimulation takes place. Intramedullary pinning, although not in itself an electrical-induced solution, may produce more piezoelectric charges across the fracture site due to pressure and possible friction due to loading. These charges causing minute currents across the fracture may cause healing to take place and appear to back up Sarmiento's [21] (1981) suggestion of pressure or slight movement at the fracture site being stimulative. This is in line with the process involved in Wolff's Law of bone deposition under stress.

With this discussion it may be that a small electric current flow achieves the same effect as natural currents. The strength of the current may be only micro-amps or less and in line with the Du-Bois measurements [5] across lesions to be ideal. These probably match the natural perineural currents. Also, it does not have to specifically be a direct current, since similar successful results have been obtained by electromagnetic induction of measurable charges into the fracture site. These charges produce small pulsed currents that appear to have the same effect as the natural ones and are now medically accepted as a possible treatment for problem fractures. Overstimulating with an enforced higher current achieved by much higher voltages, may be detrimental as other structures may be affected. Theses can include muscles and burns to the skin at the contact points. This latter effect was an occasional problem using the faradic devices to stimulate muscle growth as previously discussed.

For a veterinary therapist who may be considering using this form of stimulation to assist the healing of fractures or lesions, access may be a problem. For fractures in animal patients, the use of pins directly into the fracture segments is not an option since it is a surgical technique. This could only be carried out under operative conditions by a veterinary surgeon. There are many other considerations that need to be addressed if microcurrents are to be used, not just for fractures but for conditions thought to be suitable, such as:

1. Fractures (non-pinned connection)
2. muscle wastage
3. injury
4. slow healing lesions

Other conditions will be looked at later in this section of the book, and results drawn from research will be discussed, but some thought for the therapists to consider are specific targeting of areas that may benefit from the treatment.

In chapter seven where muscle stimulation was discussed, current from two specifically placed electrodes was said to follow the easiest path in order to form the circuit between them. The initial resistance at the contact points is reduced by using specifically designed self-adhesive pads that contain an electrically conductive gel within the adhesive. Interstitial fluid under the skin surface is a very easy path for currents to follow, so that if used for orthopaedics the application should be at the nearest position to the problem area at a point where there is very little subcutaneous fat. Bony prominences such as tuberosity's, trochanters, condyles and malleoli or along tibial plateaus being ideal attachment points.

Of course, orthopaedics is only one area where microcurrents may be applied. However, many claims are made for their efficacy, from treatment of sore muscles to headaches. In this book and others, I have made the statement that no electrotherapy actually heals any condition whether direct or inductive stimulation is applied to induce charges into tissue. The body is stimulated to initiate healing from within. If the conditions are not met naturally then therapies such as microstimulation may help replace missing charges such as perineural currents.

If the early measurements across injury sites, as suggested by Carlos Matteuci [17], are the correct value found to be flowing through lesions, then it follows that microcurrent stimulation should match these currents in order to optimise the rates of healing. This would suggest that externally applied currents need to be limited to avoid overstimulation. If taking the case of dry skin application across a lesion, then from 500,000Ω to 800,000Ω resistance may be encountered. Using a high impedance digital multimeter, two-point resistance measurements from seven volunteers produced resistance values on dry skin of between 600,000 to around 1 megaohm (1,000,000Ω). Under these conditions, the voltage levels needed to be applied across a lesion would follow the simple ratio of $V = I \times R$. where V is in Volts, I would equal 1 microamp and R, in this example, at 800,000Ω average for dry skin. Using scientific notation $V = 1 \times 10^{-6} \times 8 \times 10^{5} = 10^{-1}$ Volts. This is just 100 millivolts or one-tenth of a volt. Dampening the point of contact reduces the measured resistances significantly to resistance levels of between 300,000 to 500,000 Ω. The problem using a fixed voltage is that no two injuries or lesions are the same and from our own measurements resistance across extremities of humans, varies significantly. For a large wound many nerve endings would be severed and the exposed endings, acting as terminals, would supply a leakage current along the entire length of the wound. The problem would arise if the wound is wide, possibly due to a loss of intervening tissue. In these cases, microcurrent therapy may provide some assistance by overcoming the increased resistance across the wound. For this case higher voltages may be needed to supply the minimum required currents across the length of the lesion.

Back with orthopaedic injuries, the same logic as above would also apply to fractures, particularly compound ones, where there may be many splinters and fragments. With the natural stimulation from perineural currents, the currents would find the easiest path to an oppositely charged neurological terminal nerve created at the time of injury. This would possibly bypass most of the fracture site leading to a state of non-union.

Treatments using microcurrents

A consideration not discussed so far with microcurrents is whether pulsing or a simple direct current is the most effective. All energy transfers require some dynamic component to be effective. Direct current stimulation is a steady state current flow through tissue only moderated by the resistance encountered between the two terminals of the supply. Earlier on in this chapter perineural currents were suggested to originate from a charge difference between the two hemispheres of the brain. This would be suggestive of a constant current, varying very little. However, I would theorise that there may be a dynamic aspect to these overall direct current flows. The level of the current flow may vary but still maintain an overall unidirectional flow. The current flow could be said to be 'modulated' by other influences that may have a stimulating effect where injuries are encountered.

Low-voltage stimulation has been subjected to my own experiments using voltage ranges between 1 to 11.3Volts. It is highly unlikely that any noticeable effect would result by just connecting a small low-voltage battery to the skin via conductive self-adhesive pads. An easily measurable current can easily be proved to be established by a readily available high impedance digital multimeter. However, our experiments carried out on human volunteers showed a discernible effect felt by the volunteers at voltages from around 6+ Volts being applied when pulsed. The rates of pulses were delivered from a unit with base frequencies of 50Hz and 200Hz availability. Also, this could be gated at various rates from 5Hz to 25Hz or applied constantly. The sensations felt by the volunteers were said to be a slight sensation in the muscle. This sensation increased as the frequencies were increased. 200Hz was found to be the most effective.

The tingling sensation felt at such low voltages could be from stimulation of nerves or more likely from the muscles being caused to respond and effectively twitch at the frequency of current being passed through them. None of the volunteers expressed distress from the sensations felt. It is likely that the pulses just slightly affect the calcium channels in the sarcoplasmic reticulum causing them to release very small amounts of calcium into the sarcomere affecting just a very small number of sarcomeres. This causes a small but discernible sensation from a series of micro-twitches. This was discussed in depth in the previous chapter.

Applying this type of therapy to veterinary use, would require assessment of the suitability of the injury presented. Where there are injuries to limbs resulting in atrophy of the muscles, the early stages may be helped by low voltage pulsed stimulation. This very low series of twitches may help keep the muscle conditioned without undue stress being applied. Like all direct contact-therapy, the need for training is required and such training should highlight the benefits of each therapy and how they can be used in conjunction with other types along with the more familiar physical therapies. Low voltage stimulation may well be included as a preconditioning therapy before more pro-active ones are applied.

Discussion

With cuts and lesions, low voltage therapy may be a useful adjunct dependent on other conditions presented. With infections and debrided tissue, these need veterinary intervention and applying direct electrostimulation therapy is not recommended until the wound is consolidated. With injuries that are clear of infections and appearing to heal normally, applying an electrotherapy may not be needed as the wound will heal at its own rate. This can depend on other factors such as general heath of the animal, heart, liver lung and kidney functions, etc. Since calcium is essential for wound repair, blood circulation problems may prolong the healing phase of any lesion. In these sorts of cases, low-voltage stimulation across the wound may well add to the natural current of healing previously discussed, optimising the conditions for healing.

The photograph (Figure 26) shows the application of pulsed low-voltage stimulation along the long head of the triceps muscle. No observable twitch or discomfort was noted from the horse. The pads are the sticky types. With all animals the hair needs to be short and clean. The application of a small amount of electroconductive gel, put just in the centre of each pad, helps to make a good contact through the hair to the skin. At these low-pulsed voltages iontophoresis may be possible but is more associated with direct current flow.

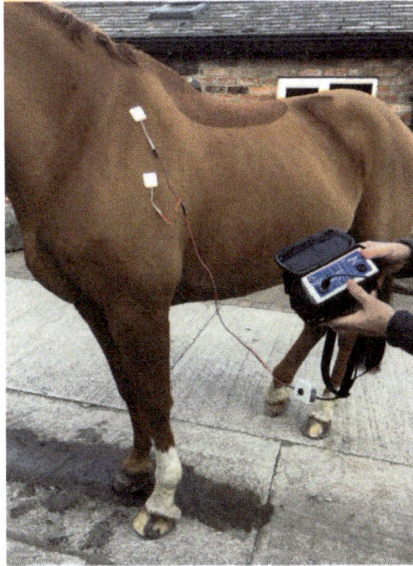

Figure 26. Low-voltage attachment. This could equally apply to high-voltage muscle stimulation

In the next chapter TENS theory and application will be discussed and how pain can be reduced by correct application. However, microcurrent therapy has had some success when researched on human patients in the area of pain reduction. A recent paper by Harikrishna and Nair [9] (2018), looked not only at the application applied to chronic wound healing but also its role in the reduction of pain. The application was to 100 patients with conditions such as diabetic foot ulcers, venous leg ulcers and pressure ulcers. Eighty-nine of the patients complained of pain. During the month-long trial all 89 reported a significant reduction in pain when microcurrents were applied across their lesions with 11 reporting that they were completely pain-free. They all showed improvements such as reduction of the lesion size and inflammatory response. Other parts of the paper confirm my belief that a pulsing microcurrent is more effective than a constant direct current. Those used in the above research suggested that a high frequency had effects on pain and the low on increasing blood flow. I would suggest high frequencies start at around 200Hz with the low ones much less at around 10 to 20Hz. This fits in with those found to be effective in pulsed magnetic therapy.

Chapter Ten

TRANSCUTANEOUS ELECTRICAL
NERVE STIMULATION (TENS)

An article by Eric L Garland [8]*(2012) defines pain as "a complex, biophysical phenomenon that arises from the interaction of multiple neuroanatomic and neurochemical systems with a number of cognitive and affective processes". He further suggests that a simpler definition is given by the International Association for the Study of Pain* [11] *(2009) "Pain is an unpleasant sensory and emotional experience associated with actual or potential tissue damage or described in terms of such damage". Both these pain descriptors are correct in that pain in either humans or animals is debilitating, reducing both the quality of life and the ability to concentrate. It is divided into two type, acute and chronic. The natural protection from harm requires that the acute response to a painful stimulus is rapid to initiate a withdrawal from the problem or the cause initiating the pain. Acute pain is relatively short-lived occurring until some sort of consolidation of the injury is set in motion. The painful response that follows is chronic and it is this that is the main long-lasting feeling of mild to extreme discomfort. Since logically both chronic and acute pain from the same source cannot be perceived at the same time gives rise to the 'pain gate theory'. This suggests that there are common ascending pathways to the brain arising from specific neurological gating systems in the spine.*

The reduction of chronic pain sometimes may be helped at source by several types of electrotherapies and analgesics. With TENS chronic pain blocking in the spinal cord is the main target or a non-painful stimulation of acute pain nerves at the source of injury whilst the chronic pain is present. This chapter looks at TENS as the electrotherapy aimed specifically at chronic pain reduction that also has striking similarities to muscle contracting devices in its design as discussed in previous chapters.

TENS or **T**ranscutaneous **E**lectrical **N**erve **S**timulation, to give it its full title, is a drug free (non-pharmacologic) analgesic treatment for pain relief. It is a proven clinically researched modality, but its actual mode of operation is based on the pain gate theory. Electrical stimulation of various sorts has been used to treat a variety of painful conditions. Historically, ancient Egyptian hieroglyphs are said to depict electric eels being placed on wounds and, if true, is possibly one of the earliest form of electrotherapy. Various interpretations of the hieroglyphs suggest that they were used to treat pain. Many other claims suggesting magnets and crystals were used by the ancient Egyptians to treat pain and used by no less a person than queen Cleopatra. These are fanciful, fictitious, a marketing ploy and have no basis in historical fact. Ancient Egyptians, like the ancient Greeks who themselves are credited with discovering and naming effects that we would now classify as static charges, did not have an understanding of the use of electricity in the body. There is no evidence that Cleopatra knew of, let alone used, magnetic rocks (lodestone) in any therapeutic way. The use of electric eels *may* be the one verifiable exception but is still open to different interpretations that the serpent like fish represented on the hieroglyphs, is in fact an electric eel.

Research in the latter half of the 1990s reviewed clinical claims and scientific explanations regarding TENS. It suggested that pain reduction is not just confined to treating the spine in its application but to the peripheral nervous system also. Since most pain can arise from all parts of the body, there is a need to understand how pain originates by looking at the anatomy and physiology of pain sensors, and how they are stimulated and transmitted to the brain. An understanding of the theory of how the brain identifies and localises them is an aid to applying therapies to effectively reduce the perception of pain felt by the patient.

Ascending nerves from around a body are from proprioceptor and nociceptors. Proprioceptors determine position and location of all parts of the body and form a feedback loop to and from the brain to maintain such things as balance and spatial awareness. Sensory receptors are from nociceptors. These supply sensory information including pressure and heat and pain responses. Looking at pain receptors that transmit acute pain stimuli such as sharp pricks from plant spikes etc. or from touching a hot surface, these quickly are transmitted to the brain's cerebellum and lower thalamus areas. They then are interpreted as a threat and cause an immediate response to remove the possibility of increased or permanent injury at the stimulated site.

Certain areas of the body are more populated with sensors than others and in humans this can be represented by the 'cortical homunculus'. There are many representations and images showing this that are readily available on web searches. Fast neural pathways transmit action potentials (APs) by fully myelinated fibres through saltatory conduction. The speed that these alpha fibres transit at is up to 40mph/65kph. The E L Garland definition gives neuroanatomical and neurochemical sources as the interactive cause. All sensors have this in common.

How the brain perceives pain may be based on the intensity of stimuli. Neurons send APs around the body by a system of a membrane charge increase from the axon hillock at the start of its axon, (see figure 16). This increase reaches a voltage threshold that sends a charge change in membrane potentials as a kind of a Mexican wave along the axon. This was discussed in depth in chapter 7. The conditions for the resulting action potential depend on complex decisions based on inputs to the many dentrites attached to the neuron. With sensory nerves it is possible to view them in a similar way to a neuron. They too develop APs but, unlike decision making neurons, stimuli caused by various means generate APs transmitted from them from only one input per nociceptor.

Nociceptors are found throughout the body but more noticeably in the skin. Stimulants detected by specialising nociceptors are:

1. Mechanical (pressure),
2. Heat (thermal) and
3. Chemical.

The following are the different types of nociceptors associated with pain sensations.

Free nerve endings are 'polymodal' in that they can be stimulated by different means. Their ability to generate action potentials that are interpreted by the brain as different sensations including pain are not fully understood at the time of writing but are thought to be changes in ionic transfer affecting electrochemical membrane voltage changes at the nerve ends. These may be caused by temperature changes at both hot and cold levels and also by neurotransmitters such as prostaglandin released from injured cellular structures due to physical or mechanical shocks. Most free nerve endings are small gauge type C slow transmission unmyelinated nerves but there are fast myelinated ones more associated with acute responses from pressure and heat. The latter are transmitted by the larger fast alpha (A∂) pathways. All nociceptors communicate with the brain sending by individual 'maintenance' APs at a rate of around one per second. Temperature may reduce or increase these giving the cool or warm sensations, repectively. When stimulated with a more repetitive chain of APs, due to higher temperatures sensed, the brain recognises these as being pain signals once certain thresholds are reached. The greater number, or more rapid the chain, determines the intensity of the perception. This means that if the number arriving at the brain is extremely high then the brain will quickly interpret this as acute pain and repond by sending APs down efferent A∂ pathways to initiate the appropriate muscular withdrawal response.

The other important sensory cells are Merkel cells. Merkel or Merkel-Ranvier cells are mechanoreceptors that sense light touch and are located very superficially at the base of the epidermis of all mammals. They are slow response cells that once activated maintain the sensation of touch much longer than other sensory types that very quickly adapt. They work in conjuction with other nerves including free nerve endings. They store and, when activated, release serotonin to stimulate these nerves. Their primary function is called Piezo2 in that Merkel cells are transducers that change mechanical forces into electrochemical signals via ion conductance in specialised channels.

Pain gate theory is based upon the sharing of common pathways to the brain. This pathways sharing can easily be demonstrated by touching the central region of the back of a willing partner, with one or two fingers. Dermatome regions are superficial areas around the body where all the sensory nerves within small areas share the same sensory pathway. Touching with any number of stimuli within a single region will only be felt as one touch. Move one touch out of the region into an adjacent one will then be sensed separately as two stimuli. Another example is that pain receptors in the heart share the same pathways as those coming from the upper left arm and shoulder. A myocardial infarction (heart attack) results in painful feelings in these areas due to this sharing but originating from within the cardiac muscle.

Pain gate theory suggests that the area where neural pathways and sharing takes place and meet is in the dorsal horn of the spinal cord. Specialised neurons, called inhibiting interneurons and projection or transmitter neurons, are synapsed (chemically connected) by both fast and slow nerve fibres originating from nociceptors throughout the body. Figure 27 below is a simplified view of these nerve fibre junctions and gives rise to how the gate theory of pain works but is probably better described as 'a theory of how chronic pain can be blocked'.

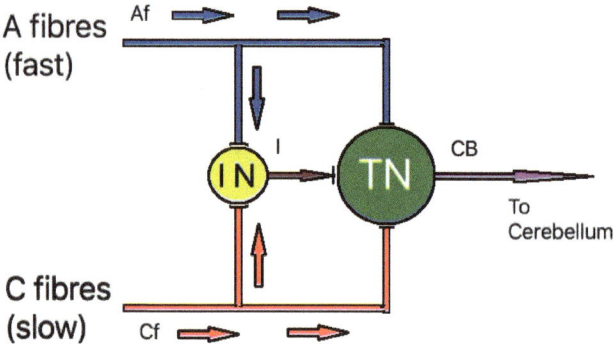

Figure 27. Simplified representation of gate theory action.

To understand the pain gate theory it is possible to model it on a simple logic circuit, see figure 28. It could be described as an 'exclusive Or gate' represented by a single 2 input device that inverts the output to '0' if two '1s' are applied at the input. However, the circuit below is more representative of the neurons and interconnections involved in the pain gate.

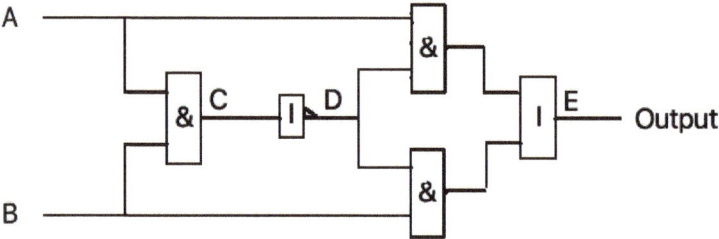

Figure 28. Logic circuit pain gate theory model

The first 2 input 'And' gate with output 'C', models the inhibitor interneuron in figure 27. This is linked via C through an invertor that turns a 1 into a zero and vice versa to provide 'D' a potentially inhibitory input to the second 2 input 'And' gates. These pair of 'And' gates feed the final 'Or' gate that collectively models the projection transmitter neuron. E is the output. All 'And' gates require that their inputs are at a logic state '1' to set the output to '1'. This '1' represents a 5-volt level in earlier computing circuits.

A logic state '0' is zero volts. The 'Or' gate will set the output to '1' if either **or** both inputs are '1s'. All logic circuits such as that shown above have a 'truth table' that predicts an output for a given set of input conditions. If A is the equivalent of the fast transmission fibre Af and B the equivalent of slow transmission Cf then the truth table shown below would be true for both the pain gate theory of interconnecting neurons (figure 27) and the modelled logic circuit (figure 28).

In the pain gate 'truth' table the interneuron is the inhibitor or control neuron equating to an 'And' gate. The TN is sometimes called the projection neuron. 'T' in my example stands for transmitter. This equates to a controlled 'Or' gate that is capable of being turned off by the interneuron input. A truth table, as mentioned above, is used in computing to predict the output of electronic gates based upon the inputs to those gates. It follows a logical binary process and may be demonstrated as below. A '1' indicates an active fibre whether slow or fast. A '0' indicates inactive.

'A' fibres transmit action potentials from specific nociceptors. This is a rapid chain of action potentials caused by harmful stimuli directly applied to the sensory nociceptor and is also capable of causing cellular damage. Provided there are no inhibiting factors, these transit the pain gate unimpeded and are recognised by the brain as acute pain signals eliciting an immediate response to try to mitigate the source of the injury. These acute pain signals are of relatively short duration compared to the chronic pain signals sent along slow unmyelinated pathways from pain receptors. These are stimulated by specific neurotransmitters released from damaged cells and are typically part of the prostanoids group and histamines released from damaged cells.

In rare cases where both chronic APs are transmitted at the same time as the acute, possibly due to a double trauma at the same site, a period may occur when pain is greatly reduced due to both fast and slow fibres being active at the pain gate. As the stimulus for the acute pain signals ceases then the slow pain signals will be allowed to pass and perceived by the brain as chronic, nagging pain. This process can be demonstrated by applying logic circuit techniques as discussed above and set in a table 3, as listed below.

Af (A fibre) 70 kmph	Cf (C fibre) 6.5 kmph	I (Interneuron) (GABA)	Cb (To brain)
0 (inactive)	0 (inactive)	0 (inactive)	0 (inactive)
1 (active)	0 (inactive)	0 (inactive)	1 (active)
0 (inactive)	1 (active)	0 (inactive)	1 (active)
1 (active)	1 (active)	1 (active)	0 (inactive)

Table 3. Pain gate theory truth table

The above table shows that the control of the transmitter/projection neuron is from the interneuron. GABA, gamma-Aminobutyric acid (γ-Aminobutyric acid) is a neuro- transmitter formed in certain neurons and, in this case, interneurons, and transported in vesicles via microtubules within the axon. These synapse with the transmitter/projector neuron. Action potentials generated by the interneuron are caused by the Alpha and C type nerves synapsing with it at the same time. They are then transmitted along its short axon to the transmitter neuronal synapse. This causes GABA channels at the presynaptic side to release the GABA into the cleft.

GABA receptors on the transmitter neuron detect this neurotransmitter, whose purpose is to inhibit the transmitter neuron from working, effectively shutting it down. The shared ascending pathway is effectively blocked, ceasing the sending of pain signal to be sensed by the brain. The significance for TENS in how it effectively causes the interneuron to release GABA, is that short, sharp high voltage stream of electrical charges will stimulate fast acting nerve pathways without further stimulating slow ones. The frequency and intensity of these stimulating charges is sufficient to cause alpha pathways to synthesise action potentials. These action potentials affect the interneuron at the same time as slow transmission chronic action potentials are active. The net effect is to enable the inhibiting interneuron to block the pain transmission to the brain.

There is one slight problem with the whole pain gate theory and, as with logic circuit modelling, is that of synchronisation. It is known that the effectiveness of TENS devices can become reduced over time. The suggestion is that the brain begins to identify real pain signals from those unnaturally blocked by the TENS device. It suggests that some signals are getting through the pain gate. With the modelled logic circuit, the two '1s' on the inputs A and B must be present at the same time to allow an output at C that is then inverted to inhibit the other 'And' gates outputs '1s' to pass through the 'Or' gate.

In the biological system the repetition rate of 'C' fibre APs would not be in total synchronous with the TENS generated pseudo A∂ APs therefore the interneuron will not be activated unless the two input APs coincided. The rate of firing of APs by the projection neuron may, as a result, continue but be erratic and at an overall rate greatly reduced than those originating as chronic pain signals. However, an assumption can be made that the slower pain signal APs have an absolute refractory time significantly longer than those of the A∂ pathways, due to the much slower speed of transit of C pathways. This overlap of APs synapsing with the interneuron would only allow APs through the gate to the brain where a gap coincides between the slow APs that may also coincide with the fast and shorter duration APs of the A∂ pathway. This again can be modelled with logic timing as shown below in figure 29:

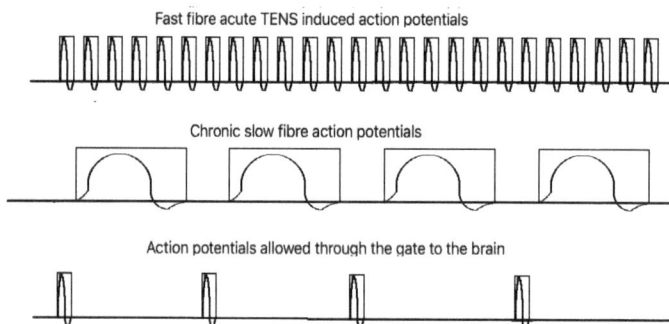

Figure 29. Gating theory of synchronous action potentials

The above diagram suggests that where absolute refractory times overlap, as shown with the logic equivalent boxes around each individual action potential, the pain gate will be closed only allowing the occasional AP through when fully clear of each other. It may be this, rather than total inhibition, that the brain recognises as a reduced chronic stimulus. This would mean that pain is not completely erradicated by TENS but made more bearable. Anecdotal reports from human application of TENS devices suggest that this is indeed the case. It may also mean that the brain begins to identify that the erractic rate of perceived chronic pain signals are false and it once again interprets the signals as increasingly chronic. This is again anecdotally reported that in many cases the initial successful pain relief is reduced over time and where long standing chronic pain has been present.

The above theory is based on the theory that the absolute refractory time of each action potential overlapping between 'A' and 'C' nerve fibres are of different durations. In reality this may not be true and a much greater overlap occurs than shown above. From my diagram, I have loosely measured the overlap at the acetocholine release points near the peaks of the two chains to arrive at the resulting projection chain.

Modelling in this way suggests that adjusting the frequency output from a TENS device to try to give some near synchronous would be probably more effective in blocking pain signals to the brain. It could be suggested that the lowering of the stimulus pulses from the TENS device to match the natural frequency arising from chronic pain sources may be more effective in blocking them. The APs that are allowed through the gate may match the frequency of very low chronic APs at the gaps between them. These APs are very short duration acute ones and because of the very low rate arriving at the brain, it may interpret them as 'maintenance' APs.

It is known that there are other effects from both high and low frequency TENS devices. Research by Bjordal 3 (2007) suggested that low frequency falls in the range of 1 to 8 Hz and high frequency from 25 – 150Hz where each pulse generates a maximum current of around 150mA. The ∂-opioid and receptors have, from research sources, been identified as being affected by high frequency voltage pulses and μ-opioid ones from low-frequency pulses. However the research source by Josimari DeSantana 13 (2008) is comprehensive but does not explain how exactly the high voltage or low pulses from TENS interact with these receptors. It may be that these receptors generate their own action potentials due to forced ionic activity created by the series of high frequency and high-voltage pulses applied across them. Different opioid receptors may have different thresholds with the μ types being lower than the ∂ ones. The effect of these receptors being blockaded may help in the relaxation of muscles which may also assist in the reduction of pain especially in the case of hyperalgesia.

Identifying sources of pain signals may be difficult in many respects as the perceived pain may originate from different part of the same neural pathway. Think of a hosepipe, where a blockage or twist in the pipe may reduce pressure or completely cut it off. Observing the pipe from one end would not necessarily reveal where the blockage has occurred, but the effect would be the same no matter where along the length of the pipe that the restriction is caused. If there is pressure put upon the spine due to an accident causing chronic pain, identifying specifically where the pressure is occurring may be easier to locate and this can then be a targeted area for attachment for the TENS leads across the area. If there is pain originating in the legs, then identifying the ascending nerve route into the spine may be a suitable attachment point. The dorsal root ganglia contain many chemical synapses with nerves coming from the peripheral nervous system. However, the gating system is located distally within the spinal cord.

If a TENS device is connected across a potentially painful site and the output voltage pulses are set too high, the sensation may be perceived as pain due to the pain gate allowing any externally generated action potentials through unimpeded if no chronic signals are present. If these match the pattern the brain interprets as acute, then a painful reaction may be met by an appropriate physical response by a withdrawal from the perceived area of stimulation. It follows that for any application the treatment should start with very low settings increasing slowly to a tolerable level. With humans this is easy but with animals recognising how they communicate between what is and isn't tolerable is down to the experience of the therapist. Another aspect to consider with animals is that where a chronic pain has been reduced by an electrotherapy application, the patient may not be sufficiently healed to allow full mobilisation of any affected limb. A perception that the pain has been reduced may lead the animal to over extending themselves and lead to possible injury further delaying the natural healing progress.

TENS Application Techniques

Application to small animals would require the target area to have the fur cut very short. Application of an electrical coupling gel would then connect the pad to the skin through the remaining hair. In the ideal situation the pad should be in contact with the skin.

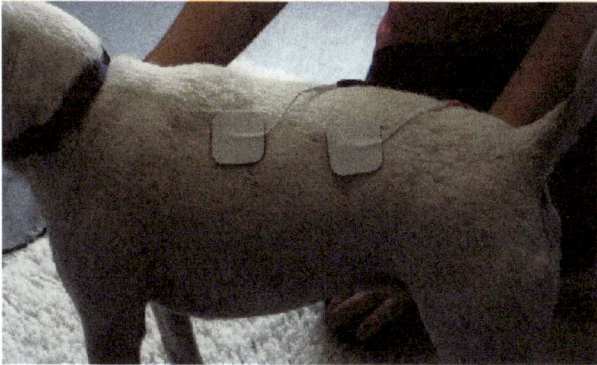

Figure 30. TENS application alongside of the spinal cord also possibly used as a muscle stimulator (single channel)

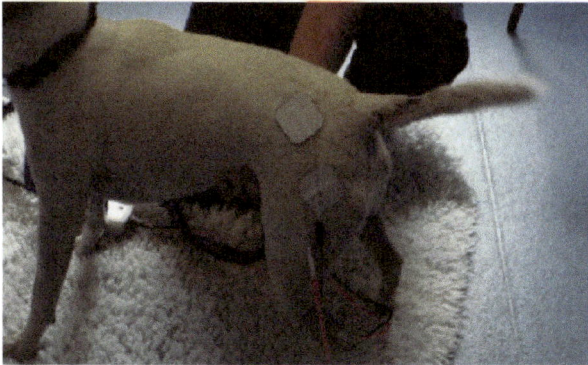

Figure 31. TENS applied to the hip muscles

Some TENS devices may have multiple channels. These allow simultaneous applications from electrically isolated pairs of output leads. This means that any one channel cannot provide a return path through the connections of an unpaired channel, only the paired channel allows a return pathway. Different manufacturers offer guidance as to how TENS devices should be connected. The following are some guidelines generalised from various sources.

Soft tissue sources of chronic pain:
- Identify the source of the pain. Check for tenderness and if possible mark the area.
- Always separate the two pads from the same channel by at least 2 inches/10cm. Never allow the pads to be in contact.
- If the source and area of the pain is identified, then the pads can be connected at opposite sides of the injury providing that there is the 10cm separation.
- Never allow the pads to be widely separated beyond the localised region of the pain source. The effectiveness is reduced by the separation distance.
- Since the pads are placed to stimulate alpha nerves specifically in a painful area, there is no hard and fast rule as to the orientation of the connections provided sufficient separation between them is maintained. Applying the pads in a way that is the most comfortable and convenient, may be adopted.

Treating orthopaedic sources of chronic pain:
Security of the positioning of the pads is an essential consideration where movements are likely to occur. These are typically over the major joints such as knee, elbow, wrists, ankles etc. both with human and equivalent animal application.

- Never place a pad where the skin surface undergoes stretching as a normal part of its function. This could be directly over or very close to a major joint. Most pads in current use are self-adhesive. Significant movement may cause the pad to lose some of this stickiness, reducing its the electrical connectivity and effectiveness, or becoming detached.
- Where a joint is the source of chronic pain, it is more effective to connect to softer tissue that may be located around the joint considering the above points about stretching.
- Never place a pair of pads alongside sources of pain. To be the most effective they must be directly across it. If incorrectly applied the stimulating currents may simply bypass the region.

Pain sensitivity over larger areas

The distance between the application of TENS pads may reduce the effectiveness as a function of the distance between them. Remember that increasing the distance between them also increases the resistance thus reducing the current for a fixed voltage setting. Where there are extended regions of pain, typically sciatic pain, then there is usually a focal point where the nerve is trapped or under pressure. This may be difficult to identify, therefore application along the length of the painful area may require the pads to be placed at the extremities. This may be even more difficult to assess in animals exhibiting signs of trapped nerve pain.

Pain originating from injury to larger muscles may present a problem alluded to in the introduction to this chapter. If the source of pain is highly localised, then applying the applicators laterally as close as possible across the muscle is required. If applied along the muscle the high voltage nature of the TENS pulses may elicit a series of twitches or even a contraction of the muscle. This similarity between muscle stimulators and TENS devices is often exploited by therapist as serving a dual purpose. However, using a TENS device as a muscle stimulator on large animals may be a little ambitious. It may help to condition an injured muscle without too much stress being applied to the whole targeted group.

TENS discussion

There are many scientific papers that back up the claim that TENS application for the reduction of pain is more than just a theory. However, the gait theory of pain reduction is still currently just that, a theory. However, as with most theories, when certain practical facts fit then acceptance follows and, like well-established theories in physics, sets of rules can be applied that work well and fit in with the theory. Looking through research papers, the one thing that is often repeated is the stimulated release of GABA, gamma-Aminobutyric acid (γ-Aminobutyric acid). This fits in well with the gate theory.

A research paper already mentioned earlier in this chapter covers mainly human responses to treatment but then reports their research using rats as subjects. A paper by Vance [26](2014) reviews much of the research to that date on the mechanisms of pain reduction. This offers confirmation from research that the main effect of TENS is on the large diameter alpha afferent nerve fibres that cause a blockade of pain transmitted signals to the brain and a mitigating reaction within the central nervous system. This then affects efferent nerves as a primary response initiating a withdrawal from the source of pain stimulus. Although some research uses rats and mice with arthritic or induced painful conditions to demonstrate the efficacy of TENS, I personally question the accuracy of such results and the ethics of purposely inflicting pain to these animals. Applying TENS to animals that are naturally in pain due to a variety of conditions in general requires skilful interpretation of pain response signals from the animal to judge frequency applied, timed duration of treatment and any negative reaction that may occur. Comparative analysis transposed from human-based research provides a basis for veterinary use. Using suitable TENS devices on oneself where a painful condition exists provides the therapist with first-hand experience of the effect. It is one of the few modalities that can offer an almost instant response that can be then applied to similar conditions that may be found on animal patients.

A full review all existing research would be capable of providing much information for a book itself. For the front line practitioner knowledge of the safe use and application of TENS and other modalities sufficient for use in practice was the main aim of this book and others in the series. Research plays an important role in giving both substance and proof to the efficacy of any electrotherapy and where there is a keen interest in deeper understanding of interactions then much further reading beyond what is referenced within this book is recommended.

Chapter Eleven

CONCLUSIONS AND GENERAL DISCUSSION
ON ELECTROTHERAPIES

In this book, as in my previous ones, I have tried to give both technical and reasoned accounts of electrotherapies in general. It is to be hoped that having reached this stage of this book, a deeper understanding of the various modalities discussed within has been achieved. The choice as to whether to use an electrotherapy is of course dependent upon the preferences of the therapists for each given situation and injury rehabilitation requirement, also a consideration for the professional therapist is the frequency of treatments that need to be applied. A one-off treatment, with the possible exception of shockwave therapy and to some extent pain reduction using TENS, is unlikely to be sufficient to keep the chronic healing phase optimised or pain reduced enough to be maintained without further intervention if other factors may inhibit or slow down natural healing processes. The frequency and timing of treatment for any regime, comes largely from experience as does the ability to discern scientific facts from the pseudo-scientific ones especially where the purchase of equipment is involved. This final chapter is very much a personal point of view that is, to some extent, based on my recent dealings with 'snake oil' salesmen, many who believe their own sales propaganda and try to pass their wares off as equivalent to genuine electrotherapy equipment produced from evidence based scientific research findings.

Readers, both therapists and pet owners should be aware that technical-sounding explanations abound for therapies that are pseudo-scientific nonsense and are sometimes associated with genuine electrotherapies. Typical of these is confusion between magnet therapy using static or permanent magnets and pulsed electromagnetic therapy. Only one of these is evidence based and empirically proven. Anything associated with a static or permanent magnet as a therapy is a scam as is their claim to induce microcurrents into tissue. The only static magnet of real use is not therapeutic but diagnostic. The extremely strong field is generated by supercooled conductivity in closed continuous coils formation in an MRI scanner. It only affects the alignment of otherwise randomly aligned hydrogen molecules and has no therapeutic value. Whilst it is not in my nature or the specific purpose of this book to publicly shame those that make and peddle scam devices, looking at a common-themes may help discriminate between fact and fiction for both direct electrical contact and static 'inducing' ones.

Claims of proof from research is ploy of many a snake oil salesperson, given that his or her target victims are never likely to question or look up such research. Proponents of non-powered devices suggest they are equivalent, or equal to electrical stimulation therapies discussed so far. They claim to be able induce minute currents into tissue. A plethora of devices are peddled as alternative therapies and magnets are at the core of most of these scams. They come as jewellery, leg wraps, collar bands, mattresses, etc. Also, there is the phenomena of the 'King's new clothes' effect in that people look to see anything that might be and improvement including natural healing progressions that they would have not closely scrutinised before putting a scam device on or around the animal. They then give undeserved credit to the device or collar. This occurs especially after purchasing such devices and reading about alleged success stories from others and, of course, proliferated by the makers. Attitudes and an eagerness to look for improvements in a beloved pet and then attributing any improvement to a scam device is a form of 'transfer placebo psychology' transferred from the owner/therapist to the animal. Animals respond to kindness, moods and to some extent, expectations of the owners, far more than people give them credit for.

Some powered direct contact therapies claiming to be able to cure anything from lung and liver cancers also are included in this assessment. It has been my recent experience that a friend and neighbour, in the terminal stages of lung and liver cancer, had bought for him a device said to pass currents through the body that could possibly cure or stop the spread of cancer. The device, sent for from outside of the UK, was expensive, large and useless. It was acquired in desperation by a loving wife wanting to try anything thought possible after reading the adverts and endorsements. Needless to say, it had no effect and he died soon after. All of the information was based on customer reviews as I could not find any research that backed up the manufacturers claims.

Another device I would strongly suggest caution over before purchase are biofeedback types. The play on the word biofeedback may sound feasible in general terms as the body is full of examples of biological feedback mechanisms that are essential to maintain homeostasis. Both negative and positive feedback takes place as part of the normal cycle and function of the body. Positive feedback is found in the production of oxytocin that increasingly induces the contractions in childbirth. The so-called theory behind these electronic biofeedback devices is that the electrical nature of the body provides noise that is detectable at the skin surface.

Nobody would doubt that such noises exist in that electrocardiograms (ECGs) and electroencephalograms (EEGs) detect pulses from the heart and brain noises at the skin surface, respectively. This includes detectable nerve stimulation. These signals can be analysed to investigate problems from identifiable rhythms and activities within the heart, brain and electrostimulation measuring nerve conduction. Biofeedback device proponents claim that all organs in the body give out specific or unique noises or frequencies that are included within surface detected noise. The claim is that subtle changes occur in the noise detected if an organ is malfunctioning. The equipment used detects the noise picked up from the skin surface. It is then amplified, inverted electronically and simultaneously fed back into the body in the belief that any affected organ or body part identifies its own contribution from the feedback noise. As it is electronically inverted, the inverted noise is applied back through the same detection electrodes. This is somehow spread throughout the body and, as it is inverted, it triggers the specific diseased organ producing the original noise to heal itself. As mentioned in an earlier chapter this is pseudo-scientific and biological nonsense that goes back to similar beliefs in the 19th century, later dismissed as the 'time of great or golden age of quackery'. Equally inverting and simultaneously feeding back any noise signal in this way would totally cancel out the original, or if fed back at a lower level, reduce it significantly.

I was asked to look at and endorse a biofeedback device that is as described above. It was very expensive £15,000 and with small whirring coolant fans and illuminated control display, looked and sounded impressive but the internal circuitry contained very little electronics. All results from treatments given were developed from patient anecdotes and endorsements. The practitioner had no recognisable medical, therapy or scientific qualifications and was treating people without medical referrals. I could not in any way justify giving the equipment any endorsement as it lacked scientific and medical credibility.

The universe is not a quiet place and is full of electromagnetic noises detectable by any high gain amplifier. If a radio is detuned, then a loud hiss is heard. This hissing sound originates from the electronic components within it including heat and also cosmic noise being induced into the aerial. The body is also a very good aerial demonstrated by physically touching a transistor radio's own aerial. Sometimes it increases the desired signal that the radio is tuned to but at other times it increases the hiss. Both are from noises and radio signals directly induced into the body tissue forming that same 'noise that biofeedback device proponents claim to be from within the body'. As a private pilot, I use a noise cancelling headset that detects and takes the spurious noise from within each earpiece. This is then electronically inverted and fed back as 'anti-noise' to the headset. The net effect is to cancel the background noise leaving only the desired speech signals that are separate to the noise picked from a small microphone embedded in the earpiece. This a real example of negative feedback based on noise. The same but inverted noise signal negatively adds to the background noise, thus cancelling out the original. Empirical research into this specific aspect of electro-biofeedback devices is lacking and as yet this sort of equipment is not marketed for animals.

I have included in this discussion non-instrumental biofeedback that may be confused with that discussed above. This comes under the 'mind-body' human alternative therapy group and, as is explained, from various sources, as "helping you focus on making subtle changes in your body". Bi-feedback proponents also state that ongoing researchers aren't exactly sure how such a therapy works but claiming that biofeedback promotes relaxation. Although I have yet to see any animal application of this type of therapy biofeedback, I would suggest that all relaxation techniques included in the qualified veterinary physiotherapist's inventory of skills will have the same effect and at much less cost and is proven to work.

Another device coming under the electronic biofeedback category detected at the skin surface was a device that I was asked to do some research analysis on. It started treatment by initially carrying out a two-contact bilateral recording of EEG functions believed to be detectable and taken from the mastoid process on human subjects. Functional analysis using Fourier transforms identified bands of frequencies in detected brainwaves that were lowered. This was determined from database comparisons. The theory was that various neurological conditions would affect one of the four types of pattern. These are Beta, Alpha, Theta and Delta waves. The deficiencies or lack of amplitude in the very low frequency delta waves is believed to be associated with conditions such as migraine and Myalgic-Encephalomyelitis (ME).

Once identified, a watch-type device was programmed at the exact rate of the lowered waveform frequency and specific to the patient. It then was then worn on the wrist and radiated an energetic electromagnetic pulse from an antenna directly into tissue. The theory behind this was that this induced pulse would induce a pseudo action potential into the ascending afferent nerve fibres and be detected by the brain as a regular but foreign stimulus. The suggestion was that the brain would then try to mask this frequency by negative feedback mechanisms thereby restoring the missing or lowered frequency. Analysis of the data from a clinical trial of 25 active and 25 sham devices, trialled were based on the migraine patient's recurrence scoring of frequency of attacks over several weeks was carried out. My analysis of the data showed no difference between active and sham. Both had a flashing LED indicating activity, so all patients believed their device was working and had no possible way of detecting the active devices. Both sham and active devices gave slightly positive results and so did not support claims of its value but more of a placebo effect. The company folded shortly after this trial. As an interesting follow-up to this I took EEG recordings, with the equipment provided, using similar methods to human patients, from a small horse. The bands of frequencies detected by the device were very similar to those from human patients! This suggested to me that much of the noise detected both from human subjects and the horse was more likely to be from external sources as discussed before.

In earlier chapters of this book and in each of the others, I have made the statement that no electrotherapy will actually heal any condition or injury or increase the speed of metabolism involved in healing process, but it may optimise the conditions, stimulate or initialise, as with shockwave application or quickly reduce pain. This is the same way that surgical intervention will correct specific injuries and conditions, but the healing of such injuries is carried out by the body and at its own rate. Claims that magnets, crystals, copper bracelets, reiki and many others offering 'positive energy', cyclotron effect, cellular resonance etc., are scams and can only affect the person using them because they believe they are doing some good, and in many cases because the pseudo-scientific sounding explanations seem plausible to the non-scientific mind leading to the placebo effect. Positive energy is a misleading play on words.

Energy can only exist as a potential to do work or as work being done, the latter being called kinetic energy. Again, the concept of positive or negative energy is a nonsense, as is the idea of spinning magnetic fields causing a 'cyclotron effect' from a static magnet formation. This is a scientific impossibility and I would suggest any reader looks up the in-depth science behind cyclotron generators. In humans the placebo effect is the belief that can give a feeling of well-being and, in some cases, be a stimulus to help optimise the body's own healing systems. Animals are a different case. They know nothing of the placebo effect and as has been pointed earlier, respond to kindness and attitude causing improvements that are then often attributed to scam therapies being applied.

Summing up the role of the electrotherapies discussed in this book.
For the new entrants into the veterinary physiotherapy profession, low current, direct contact electrical stimulation therapies offer a cost-effective way in to equipment ownership. TENS devices are easily purchased at well-known pharmacies and are relatively cheap to buy. Training in the use of such therapies should have been included on good university accredited and run courses.

Ultrasound is a different matter requiring a certain amount of specialisation. However, for demonstration purposes during a lecture, I purchased a shortwave ultrasound device from a pharmacy and wanted to demonstrate the effects with water in both 'atomisation' forming a water vapour mist around the head along with an underwater demonstration using Lycopodium powder sprinkled on the surface to show direction effects from the head. The applicator died as soon as it was submerged and was unrecoverable. The moral of this story is that:

1. always read the instructions, and
2. for professional use, always go for a rugged well-established device that states that it can be used underwater.

The pharmacy supplied one was much cheaper but as the demonstration demonstrated, not built for all the potential applications likely to be encountered by the therapist.

Before applying any electrotherapy and especially the ones covered in this book, the suitability of the patient, conditions presented, and the ability and skill required to treat are paramount. Using an electrotherapy device just because it is available should not override the suitability of the condition to be treated by any modality conveniently to hand. Whilst many of the therapies discussed are relatively benign with few contraindications, applying one that is known to have no effect for a given condition, is unprofessional but may satisfy some less enquiring owners, convincing them that their animal is receiving treatment. As mentioned earlier, however, the ability to justify and explain the application and effects in both biological and scientific terms without resorting to falsehoods, is far more satisfying. In this day and age, many owners are more enquiring and technically savvy. It is hoped that my writings in this and my previous books have helped prepare professional therapists for any such eventuality.

David Somerville 2018, email: drdcsomerville@gmail.com

References

The following list includes references used in this book. It is not exhaustive and further reading can be found on ResearchGate covering papers on the modalities discussed in this book.

1. American Heart Foundation. Penetration and attenuation of 40kHz ultrasound in animal tissue. Retrieved from: https://vct-clcctrotherpy. co.uk/40-kHz-ultrasound-penetration.php
2. Becker R., Selden G (1985) **The Body Electric: Electromagnetism and the Foundations of Life**. Pub HarperCollins.
3. Bjordal et al (2007) Short term efficiency of physical interventions of osteoarthritic knee pain. A systematic review and meta-analysis of randomised placebo-controlled trials. BMC Musculoskeletal Disorder; 8-51.
4. Bradnock, Law HT, Roscoe K. (1996) A Quantitative Comparative Assessment of the Immediate Response to High Frequency and Low Frequency Ultrasound ('Longwave Therapy') in the treatment of Acute Ankle Sprains, Physiotherapy, Volume 82, Pages 7-84 B
5. Du-Bois-Reymond Retrieved from https://www.britannica.com/ biography/Emile-Heinrich-Du Bois Reymond
6. Dyson M. (1987) Mechanisms involved in therapeutic ultrasound. Physiotherapy 73(3) 116-120 January 1987.
7. Frez A.R. (2006). Effect of Effect of continuous therapeutic ultrasound in rabbit growth plates. www.scielo.br/pdf/rbme/v12n3/en_v12n3a08
8. Garland E L (2012) Prim Care. 2012 Sep: 39(3) 561-576

9. Harikrishna KR Nair MD FMSWCP, May 2018, Microcurrent as an adjunct therapy to accelerate chronic wound healing and reduce patient pain. *Journal of Wound Care*.

10. Hyperphysics.phyastr.gsu.edu/hbase/Sound/usound2.html Speed of sound in tissue.

11. International Association for the Study of Pain (2009) retrieved from: https://en.wikipedia.org/wiki/International_Associationfor the Study of Pain

12. Journal of Ultrasound in Medicine. Retrieved from onlinelibrary.wiley.com/doi/10.7863/jum.2011.30.1.21/full

13. Josimari DeSantana et al. (2008) Effectiveness of Transcutaneous Electrical Nerve Stimulation for treatment of Hyperalgesis and Pain. Curr, Rheumatol. Rep 2008 Dec. (6): 49– 499.

14. Laycock (Somerville) D C. (1991) Vibrational Analysis of Fracture Healing in Long Bones. PhD thesis, University of Salford Department of Orthopaedic Mechanics.

15. Lehmann J.F, Herrik JF. (1953) Biological reactions to cavitation, a consideration for ultrasound therapy. ARCH Phys Med Rehab 1953; 34:86-98.

16. Levine David, Millis Darryl L. Veterinary Surgery (2001), Effect of 3.3MHz on Caudal Thigh Muscle Temperature in Dogs. University of Tennessee, Knoxville.

17. Matteuci Carlos. References can be found at www.britannica.com/biography/Carlo-Matteucci

18. Nicholas D, 1982, Evaluation Backscatter coefficients for excised human tissues: Results, interpretation and associated measurements. Ultrasound in Medicine & Biology 8(1): 17-28

19. Notamicola et al (2014) Chel therapy in the treatment of chronic insertion

Achilles tendinopathy. *Lasers Med Sci* 2014:29:1217-25.

20. Rompe JD et al (2005) Repetitive low-energy shock wave application without local anaesthesia is more efficient than repetitive low-energy shock wave with anaesthesia in the treatment of chronic plantar fasciitis. J Orthop. Res2005:23:931-41.

21. Sarmiento A, Latta L (1981) Close functional treatment of fractures. Springer-Verlag: Heidelberg.

22. Schmitz C.et al : PEDro database' (2015) A review of the studies found in the PEDro Database. Retrieved from https://www.**pedro**.org.au

23. Smith T. et al: (2004) The microvascular and hemodynamic mechanisms for the therapeutic actions of H-Wave muscle stimulation. Orthopaedic Surgery, Wake Forest University School of Medicine, Winston-Salem, NC.

24. Tascioglu F, Kunzin D, Armagan O and Ogutler G (2010) Short -term Effectiveness of Ultrasound Therapy in Knee Osteoarthritis. *The Journal of International Medical Research* 2010; 1233-1242

25. Retrieved from https://standards.globalspec.com/std/530143/bsi-**bs-5724-1**

26. Vance C et al. (2014) Using TENS for pain control: the state of evidence, Pain Manag. 2014 May: 4(3):197-209.

27. WOMAC Index (1982) www.womac.org/womac/index htm